CONSCIOUS-SEDATION IN DENTAL PRACTICE

CONSCIOUS-SEDATION IN DENTAL PRACTICE

C. Richard Bennett, D.D.S., Ph.D.

Professor and Head, Department of Anesthesiology, and
Professor, Department of Pharmacology and Physiology,
University of Pittsburgh School of Dental Medicine; Professor,
Graduate School (Dental Medicine), University of Pittsburgh;
Associate Professor, Department of Anesthesiology, University of
Pittsburgh School of Medicine; Staff Anesthesiologist and Chief of Dental
Services, Presbyterian-University Hospital, Pittsburgh, Pennsylvania;
Consultant Staff, Children's Hospital, Eye and Ear Hospital, Magee-Women's Hospital,
Montefiore Hospital, and Leech Farm Veterans Administration Hospital,
Pittsburgh, Pennsylvania

SECOND EDITION

with 99 illustrations

The C. V. Mosby Company

SAINT LOUIS   1978

SECOND EDITION

Copyright © 1978 by The C. V. Mosby Company

All rights reserved. No part of this book may be reproduced
in any manner without written permission of the publisher.

Previous edition copyrighted 1974

Printed in the United States of America

The C. V. Mosby Company
11830 Westline Industrial Drive, St. Louis, Missouri 63141

Library of Congress Cataloging in Publication Data

Bennett, Charles Richard, 1938-
  Conscious-sedation in dental practice.

  Bibliography: p.
  Includes index.
  1. Anesthesia in dentistry. 2. Sedatives.
I. Title. [DNLM: 1. Anesthesia, Dental.
2. Hypnotics and sedatives. WO460 B471c]
RK510.B4   1978   617′.967′6   78-4565
ISBN 0-8016-0612-8

C/CB/B   9   8   7   6   5   4   3   2   1

CONTRIBUTORS

Kay F. Thompson, B.S., D.D.S.

Assistant Professor, Department of Behavioral Sciences,
University of Pittsburgh School of Dental Medicine;
Continuing Education Faculty, University of Pittsburgh
School of Dental Medicine, Pittsburgh, Pennsylvania;
Fellow and President of the American Society of Clinical and Experimental
Hypnosis; Associate Editor, American Journal of Clinical Hypnosis;
Associate Member and Fellow, American Society of
Clinical and Experimental Hypnosis

Robert E. Pearson, M.D.

Assistant Director of Training and Research, Traverse City
State Hospital, Traverse City, Michigan; Adjunct Assistant Professor,
University of Michigan, Department of Psychiatry, Ann Arbor, Michigan;
Past-President and Fellow, American Society of Clinical and Experimental Hypnosis;
Associate Member and Fellow, American Society of Clinical and
Experimental Hypnosis

FOREWORD

Conscious-Sedation in Dental Practice details a philosophy of pain relief and safety in dental practice. Equating dental care with pain and suffering can and should now be a feature of the past. Dr. Bennett not only gives the background knowledge necessary for the practice of safe relief of pain in dental care but also uniquely introduces the dentist and dental student to evaluation of the whole patient, to recognition of systemic complications that require medical attention, and to reversal of life-threatening emergencies by resuscitative measures.

All of this reflects the author's vision and his public health orientation. He agrees that the medical and dental professions must place a high priority not only on reducing but also on entirely abolishing the deaths and crippling complications caused by anesthesia. I believe that many of the philosophies espoused in this text will promote this goal.

Exact data on anesthesia-related mortality do not exist. Among about 20 million surgical anesthetics given each year in the United States, an estimated 3,000 lead to death of the patient, with anesthesia management being primarily at fault; in several thousand more, anesthesia has been a contributing factor in the patients' demise. Although the estimated incidence of death associated with dental anesthesia is lower, some healthy persons still are dying as a result of local or general anesthesia that are used for dental procedures that are not essential for survival. They die from airway obstruction, respiratory depression, circulatory depression, or convulsions as the result of inept management of the anesthesia and/or resuscitation or from other unfortunate circumstances. Conscious-sedation preserves upper airway protective reflexes, patient cooperation, and integrity of circulation and thus avoids the dangers of general anesthesia, while the single operator can produce pain-free dental work, even in patients with emotional disorders. Safety is the prime motif of this book.

Every dentist can and should learn these techniques, as has been shown by the vast experience at the University Health Center of Pittsburgh. The student must realize, however, that learning these artistic combinations of regional analgesia and conscious-sedation requires more than book knowledge. It is an art that is acquired through supervised introductory experience and long-term practice. This approach of conscious-sedation is one of several examples in medical and dental care of replacing the prevalent cookbook approach of "treatment by prescription" with the physiological approach of "treatment by titration." Although many different drugs and routes of administration are described here, the student should appreciate the fact that extensive experience with use of one or two of them may give better and safer results than polypharmacy based on theoretical indications.

The pathophysiology of pain is also discussed in this book. In comparison with acupuncture and hypnosis, which recently have aroused renewed interest, the titrated pharmacological conscious-sedation plus regional analgesia described here is a more reliable and quicker and thus more practical approach.

I want to conclude this foreword with a tribute to my friend and former colleague, Dr. Leonard M. Monheim, whose life work inspired this book. After his painful death from cancer at age 60, he was succeeded at the University of Pittsburgh by the author of this book. Dr. Monheim, although trained as a dentist, became a leader in medical anesthesiology. He made lasting impressions on physicians as a safe, skillful clinical anesthesiologist for all kinds of surgical procedures, as supervisor and manager of operating room anesthesia, as teacher and humanitarian, and as promoter of sound practices. His interest in both dentistry and anesthesiology permitted him to advance the work of men who were pioneers in dental anesthesia over a hundred years before his time. He helped me in the development of the Department of Anesthesiology at the University of Pittsburgh, which has become the largest in the United States in terms of work load and manpower.

Dr. Monheim's career culminated in his appointment as Professor of Anesthesiology at the University of Pittsburgh School of Medicine and in a tribute by his peers in May, 1971, for his "outstanding contribution to the development of hospital dental and anesthesia programs and the resulting close relationship of comprehensive dental and medical care to total health."

Dr. Monheim's persistent concern for safe relief of pain in dentistry is reflected not only in his own books, *Local Anesthesia and Pain Control in Dental Practice* and *General Anesthesia in Dental Practice,* which have been revised by Dr. Bennett, but also in this text by his pupil, colleague, and successor.

The spirit, knowledge, and principles conveyed by Dr. Monheim and Dr. Bennett personally and through their textbooks confirm my conviction that not only anesthesiology but also dentistry is an integral part of the art and science of medicine.

Peter Safar, M.D.

Professor and Chairman,
Department of Anesthesiology,
School of Medicine;
Anesthesiologist in Chief,
Health Center Hospitals;
and Coordinator, Multidisci-
plinary Critical Care Medicine
Program, University of Pittsburgh

PREFACE

The writing of this text was prompted by recent advances in the fields of medicine and pharmacology, a better understanding of pain mechanisms, and a realization that greater emphasis on dental health and total patient care is placing an increasing demand on the dental profession to efficiently and effectively render dental treatment to patients with physical, psychological, and behavioral disorders. It is my belief that every dentist, as a member of the health team, must satisfy the obligation placed on him by his profession to deliver dental service to all who seek dental care. Because of advances in various medical sciences the dentist of today no longer has the "luxury" of treating only healthy patients. Practitioners see many apparently healthy patients who, in reality, are physically or emotionally compromised yet pharmacologically compensated. These individuals are deserving of special attention and care if existing conditions are not to be aggravated by dental treatment.

In this text I have attempted to present a philosophy and concept of patient care that are mutually beneficial to both patient and practitioner. The ideas expressed, procedures discussed, and techniques described are well within the scope of undergraduate dental education. They offer a safe, convenient, and pleasant alternative to general anesthesia in many cases. This is attested to by the fact that the teaching of conscious-sedation has been an integral part of the dental curriculum at the University of Pittsburgh for 15 years. During this period third- and fourth-year dental students have safely employed the principles presented in well over 12,000 cases.

Every attempt has been made to deal in concepts rather than specific techniques. I believe that in this manner the reader can gain an in-depth appreciation for conscious-sedation and patient care that will provide the flexibility and versatility necessary to fulfill the needs of individual patients and practitioners.

The concepts, principles, and philosophy expressed herein are a reflection of my close association with the late Dr. Leonard M. Monheim, whose genuine interest in the dental profession, particularly the application of pain control methodology, was aptly demonstrated in his two textbooks, *Local Anesthesia and Pain Control in Dental Practice* and *General Anesthesia in Dental Practice*. It is hoped that this volume will complement Dr. Monheim's texts and further perpetuate the ideas of the pioneer with whom I had the fortune to study and work for 10 years.

My sincere gratitude is extended by Drs. Kay F. Thompson and Robert E. Pearson for their contributions. I would also like to express my appreciation to William Brent for his excellent artwork and Dr. Edward Heinrichs for photographic assistance. Thanks are also extended to Abbott Laboratories, Fraser-Sweatman, Inc., the McKesson Company, Porter Instrument Company, Inc., and Statham Instruments, Inc., for granting permission to reproduce portions of their manuscripts or providing various photographs used in this text.

I owe a special debt of gratitude to my wife Margaret, without whose encouragement and untiring devotion this manuscript would not have been possible.

C. Richard Bennett

CONTENTS

xiii

8 THE PHARMACOLOGY OF CONSCIOUS-SEDATIVE AGENTS, 102

9 TECHNICAL CONSIDERATIONS AND ROUTES OF ADMINISTRATION, 119

10 TECHNIQUE FOR INTRAVENOUS CONSCIOUS-SEDATION, 143

CONSCIOUS-SEDATION
IN DENTAL PRACTICE

Chapter 1

PAIN

Since the beginning of time, pain has been one of man's constant tormentors. Relief from it has been sought by ingesting, injecting, or topically applying a wide variety of potions and concoctions. This real but elusive entity is often spoken of as a protective mechanism manifested when an environmental change occurs causing injury to responsive tissues.

Although each of us has experienced pain, the exact meaning of the word is difficult to define. Great variances in the painful experience exist, due in many respects to a tremendous emotional involvement. Pain is often described in a variety of terms such as "sharp, lancing, burning, dull, throbbing, or aching." In addition, it may be mild or severe, constant or intermittent, spontaneous or induced.

THEORIES ON THE NATURE OF PAIN

Not only does terminology vary in describing pain; investigators also differ in their definitions and theories of the basic nature of pain. For the past few decades the exact nature of pain has been the subject of more than a few debates and controversies. During this time two opposing theories, each with good evidence to support it, have predominated. The first of these is the specificity theory; the second and more popular is the pattern theory. Recently, a third—the gate control theory of Melzack and Wall—has been introduced, which offers some plausible solutions to those aspects of pain that are not readily explained on the basis of either the specificity or the pattern theory.

Specificity theory. In 1842 a monumental contribution by Müller postulated the doctrine of specific nerve energies, which stated that the brain can receive information about external objects only through the sensory nerves. Müller recognized only the five classic senses. He further stated that sensation is a property common to all the senses but that the kind of sensation is different for each. Thus we have the sensations of light, sound, taste, smell, and feeling or touch. Touch incorporated for him all the qualities of sensory experiences that we derive from stimulation of the body surfaces. In 1895 von Frey extended Müller's theory into the specificity theory as we know it today. von Frey proposed that there are four cutaneous modalities, each subserved by a specific type of receptor that, when stimulated, conveys the impulse for the modality it represents to a specific area of the brain over specific nerve pathways. Free nerve endings were said to be the receptors for generating painful impulses.

Free nerve endings are naked nerve fibers, mostly of the unmyelinated variety. They are present as delicate fibrous loops or long hair-like networks. These fibers are termed nociceptors and are present in all structures and organs from which pain may be elicited.

Pain is said to be conducted to the central nervous system by nerve fibers of two types. These are classified according to fiber size and the speed at which they conduct nerve impulses. The A fibers are large myelinated fibers varying in diameter from 3 to 20 μm. They conduct the fast or first pain (sharp, localized) at a rate of up to 100 meters per second. (B fibers range up to 3 μm. in diameter, conduct impulses at a rate of 3 to 14 meters per second, are confined to preganglionic autonomic fibers, and do not play a role in the conduction of painful impulses.) The C fibers are small unmyelinated nerve fibers, from 0.5 to 1 μm. in diameter, and conduct slow or second pain at a rate of 0.5 to 2 meters per second.

Each afferent nerve fiber is a separate pathway by which impulses are transmitted to the central nervous system, and each pathway is a unit unto itself. A gathering of several units—perhaps a hundred—constitutes an afferent nerve trunk. The single units that form a nerve trunk may be stimulated individually or in varying numbers until all individual fibers are affected.

Despite its apparent simplicity the theory has three facets, each representing a major assumption. The first of these, that receptors are specialized, is physiological in nature and has achieved the proportions of a genuine biological law. The remaining two assumptions, anatomical and psychological in nature, are not supported by facts.

Pattern theory. The pattern theory has been proposed as an alternative to the specificity theory. This theory states that receptors are specialized physiologically for the transduction of particular kinds and ranges of stimuli into patterns of nerve impulses rather than modality-specific information. Both spatial and temporal summations of the coded impulses may occur, which allow the brain to distinguish and identify the stimulus being applied.

A painful experience may result either from summation of many simultaneous nonpainful stimulus applications or from excessive stimulation in terms of both the number of responding fibers and the frequency of impulses per fiber. This theory does not postulate the existence of a specific pain receptor.

Gate control theory. Briefly stated, the gate control theory postulates that

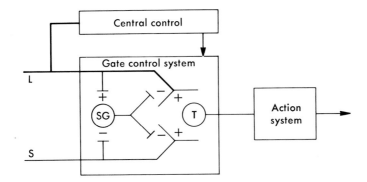

Fig. 1-1. Diagrammatic representation of the gate control theory of pain.

(1) the substantia gelatinosa of the spinal cord, which consists of small and densely packed cells, acts as a gate control system that modulates the synaptic transmission of nerve impulses from peripheral fibers to central transmission (T) cells; (2) afferent patterns in the dorsal column system of the spinal cord act, in part at least, as a central control trigger, activating selective brain processes that influence the modulating properties of the gate control system; and (3) T cells activate neural mechanisms comprising the "action system" that is responsible for perception and response (pain reaction).

Input to the T cells is via both large- and small-diameter nerve fibers that also project to the substantia gelatinosa. An inhibitory effect exerted by the substantia gelatinosa in afferent fiber terminals is increased by activity in large fibers and decreased by activity in small fibers. Thus the gate for nerve transmission from the periphery to T cells is opened by small-fiber activity and closed by activity in large fibers. This is accomplished by either presynaptic facilitation or inhibition (Fig. 1-1).

Activities and stimuli that activate large fibers (presynaptic inhibition and closing of the gate) better enable an individual to tolerate pain. Such stimuli include vibration and scratching, among others, and will be discussed later.

THE DUAL NATURE OF PAIN

Regardless of the exact mechanism involved and realizing full well that any definition is open to question, let me here define pain as an unpleasant sensation created by a noxious stimulus that is mediated along certain nerve pathways to the central nervous system, where it is interpreted as such. Examination of this definition reveals the dual nature of pain. The first aspect, or *pain perception,* is the physiologicoanatomical process by which pain is received and transmitted by neural structures to the central nervous system. The second, or *pain reaction,* is the patient's manifestation of his perception of an unpleasant experience.

Pain perception

Before there can be any pain, an environmental change in excitable tissue must take place. This change is referred to as a stimulus. It may be electrical, thermal, chemical, or mechanical in nature. The stimulus must be of a certain minimum intensity and must be applied for a certain minimum period of time in order to initiate a nerve impulse. This aspect of pain perception is referred to as the *pain perception threshold*. The intensity and duration of the threshold stimulus as well as the speed of impulse conduction can be measured, and values have been found to be remarkably similar in all individuals having healthy, intact nervous systems. The impulses, or waves of excitation, that spread along the nerve fiber are self-propagating and are of equal intensity regardless of the degree of stimulation. This is known as the all-or-none law, which simply means that a threshold stimulus (one of sufficient intensity and duration) creates an impulse as strong as, and one which is transmitted as rapidly as, that produced by a much stronger stimulus. At times this principle may seem unfounded, particularly when an exceptionally noxious stimulus applied to a nerve produces an especially great reaction. This greater response stresses the multifiber composition of the nerve. Whereas a weak stimulus affects only a few fibers, the more intense stimulus excites more (or even all) the fibers of the nerve trunk.

Regardless of the theory of pain to which one adheres, each has its strengths, weaknesses, and overlapping similarities to the others. No one of the three excludes the basic concept of the dual nature of pain. All three agree that the impulse must be initiated and transmitted to the central nervous system, and all three refer to this process as *pain perception*.

Pain reaction

Pain reaction, the second aspect of pain, embraces extremely complex neuroanatomical and physiopsychological factors involving higher nervous system centers. This phase of pain will differ from person to person and in the same person from day to day. It determines how the patient will react in response to the unpleasant experience.

Pain reaction may be defined as the patient's response to the perception process that precedes it. In the gate control theory this phase of pain is referred to as the "action system." Once the integrated and modulated firing level of the T cells exceeds a critical level, the firing triggers a sequence of response characterized in the individual by (1) a startle response, (2) a flexion reflex, (3) postural readjustment, (4) vocalization, (5) orientation of the head and eyes to examine the damaged area, (6) autonomic reflexes resulting in changes in vital signs, (7) evocation of past experience in similar situations and prediction of the consequences of the stimulation, and (8) many other patterns of behavior aimed at diminishing the sensory and affective components of the whole experience—rubbing of the damaged area, avoidance behavior, and so forth.

It is thought that the concept of a "pain center" in the cerebral cortex, as included in the specificity theory, is inadequate to account for such complex sequences of behavior. The thalamus, limbic system, hypothalamus, brainstem reticular formation, parietal cortex, and frontal cortex have all been demonstrated to take part in pain reaction.

Once again, however, regardless of the pain theory accepted, each recognizes the second phase of pain, *pain reaction.*

It is now firmly established that stimulation of the brain activates descending efferent fibers, which can influence conduction at the earliest synaptic levels of the somesthetic system. Thus it is possible for central nervous system activities subserving attention, emotion, memories of past experience, and the like to exert control over sensory input. There is evidence to suggest that these influences may be mediated through the gate control system.

Pain reaction threshold

The pain reaction threshold is commonly interpreted as being inversely proportional to pain reaction. A patient who is hyporeactive is considered to have a high pain reaction threshold, whereas a patient with a low pain threshold is hyperreactive. Consequently, reference to a patient's high or low pain reaction threshold indicates his conscious reaction to a specific unpleasant sensory experience.

Since the pain perception threshold is relatively stable but the pain reaction threshold is free to vary, the phrase "pain threshold," in its truest interpretation, depends not on pain perception but is, rather, correlated with pain reaction. Any alterations in a patient's ability to tolerate pain will depend on the complex neuroanatomical and physiopsychological factors governing pain reaction.

The following factors have been shown to have a definite bearing on a patient's pain reaction threshold.

Emotional state. An individual's pain threshold will to a great degree depend on his attitudes toward the procedure, the operation, and the surroundings. As a rule, the patient who is emotionally unstable will have a low pain threshold. It has also been observed that a patient who is greatly concerned or who has problems—not necessarily related to the dental problem at hand—also tends to have a low pain threshold. An emotionally unstable individual may have pain preception properties within the range shown by stable individuals, whereas his pain reaction is greatly increased.

Fatigue. Of significant importance to the patient's pain threshold is fatigue. The patient who is well rested and has had a good night's sleep prior to an unpleasant experience will have a much higher pain threshold than the individual who is tired and worn. It is essential that, whenever possible, a good night's sleep precede any potentially trying experience.

The dentist should acquaint himself with those agents that may be prescribed to ensure his patient a restful night before the dental office visit. Psychological and physical preparation for pain-free and apprehension-free dentistry must be initiated well in advance of the operative dental appointment.

Age. As a general rule, older individuals tend to tolerate pain and thus have a higher pain threshold than younger individuals or children. Perhaps an advanced philosophy of living or the realization that unpleasant experiences are a part of life may account for this fact. In cases of extreme age or senility, pain perception itself may be affected.

Sex. Contrary to the thoughts expressed by advocates of the Women's Liberation Movement, it is generally considered that men have a higher pain reaction threshold than women. This is, in all probability, a reflection of man's desire to maintain his feeling of superiority. This is exhibited in his predetermined effort to tolerate pain.

Fear and apprehension. In practically all cases, the pain threshold is lowered as fear and apprehension mount. Individuals who are extremely fearful or apprehensive of a procedure tend to magnify within their own minds the unpleasant experience. Such patients become hyperreactive and will magnify the pain out of all proportion to the original stimulus. It is essential, therefore, that the operator attempt to secure each patient's confidence. My experience has been that patients appreciate the dentist's interest in them and fare much better when the treatment that is to be performed is explained to them. This aids in alleviating fear and apprehension by demonstrating the dentist's concern for their welfare while under his care. This procedure has been particularly helpful in managing children.

Past experience. A patient's past experience is capable of modifying that individual's ability to tolerate pain. Those persons who have had unpleasant experiences in a dental office in the past are either consciously or subconsciously expecting pain to be associated with all dental procedures—regardless of the nature of the procedure. The practitioner must determine the nature of previous dental experiences and prepare himself and the patient appropriately. Those patients who have had pain-free dental treatment previously will generally be less fearful and apprehensive of the present dental visit.

Drugs. Various drugs can be used to alter the pain reaction. Certain agents have the ability to elevate the pain threshold at a central nervous system level, through an analgetic effect that is primarily exerted on the thalamus and cerebral cortex. Narcotic analgetics fall into this category. In addition, they can cause the patient to be a calmed or euphoric one who has a freedom from fear and apprehension. Therefore these agents may alter the pain reaction by controlling emotional and psychological factors as well.

Still other agents possess the ability to lower the pain threshold, thus rendering the patient less able to tolerate pain. Barbiturates are noted for this effect. The administration of a barbiturate in the presence of pain is unwise.

However, if pain perception is controlled (as with regional analgesia), the sedative effect of these drugs may alter the patient's emotional status in such a way that he can better cope with an otherwise trying situation.

Psychosedative agents are not, per se, capable of either elevating or lowering the pain threshold. However, their ability to potentiate other agents plus their ability to allay fear and apprehension make them valuable adjuncts in the control of pain reaction.

CONTROL OF PAIN

One of the most important aspects of the practice of dentistry is the control or elimination of pain. In the past, pain has been so closely associated with dentistry that the words "pain" and "dentistry" have become almost synonymous. Studies by the National Institute of Dental Research (1970) have shown that fear of pain makes more patients fail to seek dental treatment than do all other reasons combined. This should no longer be a fact, as pain and fear of pain can be controlled or eliminated in all phases of dental practice.

Pain in many instances is considered a necessary element of everyday living, as it is a warning of trouble. However, in the practice of dentistry, we must regard pain not as a warning signal but as an evil to be conquered.

As shown in the preceding discussion, pain may be divided into two phases, pain perception and pain reaction. Therefore any method of pain control will affect either one or both of these two dimensions.

Methods of pain control

The following are means that can be used for pain control:
1. Remove the cause.
2. Block the pathway of painful impulses.
3. Raise the pain threshold.
4. Prevent pain reaction by causing central nervous system depression.
5. Use psychosomatic methods.

Remove the cause. It is obvious that removing the cause would be a desirable method of preventing pain. If this could be accomplished, the environmental change in tissue would be eliminated and, consequently, the nerve would not be excited and nerve impulses would not be initiated. It is imperative that any removal leave no permanent environmental change in tissues, as the new condition might then be able to create an impulse even though the original causation factors had been eliminated. This method of pain control clearly affects pain perception.

Block the pathway of painful impulses. The most widely used and, without a doubt, the most important method in dentistry for eliminating pain is to block the pain pathway. By this method a suitable drug, possessing regional analgetic properties, is injected into the tissues in proximity to the nerve involved. The injected solution prevents depolarization of the nerve fiber in the area of absorption, thus preventing those particular fibers from conducting any impulses centrally beyond that point. As long as the solution is present in the nerve in sufficient concentration to prevent depolarization, the block will be in effect.

The importance of this aspect of pain control is discussed in detail in Chapter 2.

Raise the pain threshold. In recent years the dentist has become more aware of and has shown a greater appreciation for this aspect of pain control. Raising the pain threshold depends on the pharmacological action of drugs possessing analgetic properties. These drugs raise the pain threshold at a central nervous system level and thus interfere with pain reaction. In this method of pain control, the cause of the original stimulus may still be present. The neuroanatomical pathways will be intact and be able to conduct impulses. In other words, pain perception will be unaffected, but pain reaction will be decreased and thus the pain reaction threshold raised. It should be clearly understood that the pain threshold can be raised to limited degrees only, dependent on the specific drugs used. It is pharmacologically impossible to eliminate all pain that is of the most severe nature by raising the pain threshold alone. To clarify the preceding statement further, the presence of more noxious stimuli creating severe pain will necessitate either blocking the pathway of the impulse or depressing pain reaction completely, by the use of an agent that renders the patient unconscious, if pain of all degrees is to be eliminated.

Various drugs possess analgetic properties in varying degrees, and thus some are more effective in raising the pain threshold than others. Certain drugs such as aspirin (acetylsalicylic acid) are effective only in the relief of mild discomfort. On the other hand, the narcotics, though not true analgetics (because they also possess hypnotic properties), are effective against more severe pains because they are able to raise the pain threshold to a greater degree. With all drugs now used to raise the pain threshold there are optimal doses, and increasing the dosage beyond the indicated limit will not further increase the analgetic effectiveness of the drug without producing undesirable or dangerous side effects.

In addition to possessing analgetic properties, the narcotics (as well as some other, nonnarcotic agents) have the ability to allay fear and apprehension, alter the patient's mood, and better prepare the patient psychologically to accept dental treatment.

Indirectly, therefore, this beneficial effect may also aid in the control of pain by acting to close the gate mechanism, as discussed earlier, under pain reaction. The dental practitioner may take full advantage of these drugs, in combination with regional analgesia, to allow the patient to be free of operative pain, fear, and apprehension while remaining cooperative in the conscious state. Regional analgesia controls pain perception as other agents elevate the pain reaction threshold and decrease anxieties related to dental treatment.

Subsequent chapters deal with this concept in greater detail.

Prevent pain reaction by causing central nervous system depression. Eliminating pain by depression of the central nervous system is within the scope of unconscious techniques and those agents employed to render the patient unconscious. With their use, the agent of choice, by its increasing depression of the central nervous system, prevents any conscious reaction to painful stimuli. If the cerebral cortex is depressed only to the point that inhibitions are suppressed, the patient may become hyperreactive to a painful stimulus.

The use of unconscious techniques does not properly fall within the realm of the dentist who has had less than at least a year's postgraduate training and experience in its use. This particular subject has been covered in detail in another book, *Monheim's General Anesthesia in Dental Practice.*

Use psychosomatic methods. All too often the psychosomatic approach to the elimination or the control of pain is sadly neglected in dental practice. By no other method can so much be gained with so little ill effect on the patient.

This method affects only pain reaction and for its effectiveness depends on putting the patient in the proper frame of mind. It is amazing what can be accomplished without the use of drugs or as a supplement to drug therapy when the patient's faith and confidence are gained.

One of the most important factors in this approach is the use of honesty and sincerity with the patient. This necessitates keeping the patient well informed as to both the procedure and what he may expect. It is a well-known physiological axiom that the nervous system dislikes surprises and, in many instances, reacts violently toward them. The patient should be made to understand, by a kind and considerate approach, the extent of the discomfort that he may expect. Also he should be assured that any unpleasant sensory experience can be adequately controlled through the knowledge and methods at hand. Patients like to feel that their comfort and well-being are of prime concern to the dentist. Once they are secure in this feeling, they will tend to tolerate unpleasant sensations to a greater degree. It is in this manner that pain reaction is depressed and the pain threshold inversely raised. The possible role of emotional status in controlling the gate mechanisms has been discussed previously. The role of suggestion will be discussed in detail in Chapter 5.

•   •   •

Of the five methods available for the control of pain, four are within the scope of general dental practice and the scope of this text. Detailed discussions that follow will demonstrate how a combination of regional analgesia, psychosedation, analgesia as produced with nitrous oxide or narcotics, and suggestion can be combined to provide both patient and operator with the parameters required for a relaxed and productive dental appointment.

Chapter 2

THE SPECTRUM OF PAIN CONTROL

Not many years ago the practicing dentist had but two methods of pain control at his disposal. The first method, local anesthesia, was satisfactory for the majority of patients who sought dental care. Those patients not amenable to the use of this method of operative pain control were automatically candidates for the second method available, general anesthesia.

As recently as the mid-1930s the use of local anesthesia was considered unwise for patients who were undergoing any dental treatment not involving oral surgery. Even today many patients and a few dentists are still firm in this belief. Indeed, each practitioner can recall several patients in his practice who refuse local anesthesia for routine dentistry and tolerate the procedure quite well without it. Needless to say, these patients are in the minority.

The fact that pain-free dentistry was accomplished only when surgery was performed caused many potential patients to avoid routine dental care. Patients neglected oral health until their condition deteriorated to such an extent that pathological pain forced them to seek assistance. The stigmatic relationship between *pain* and *dentistry* remains with the dental profession today to the extent that the greater percentage of our population who fail to seek dental care do so out of *fear of pain*.

Better understanding of pain mechanisms, psychology, pharmacology, and related sciences has led to the development of a *spectrum of pain control,* which is well recognized and accepted by the modern dental practitioner (Fig. 2-1). The spectrum spans all methods of pain control, ranging from regional analgesia alone to general anesthesia and the production of unconsciousness. All methods are applicable to dental practice; some require specialized and extensive training, whereas others may be learned and used with safety after less involved courses of study.

Discussion will not include treatment of those patients who satisfactorily tolerate routine operative dental pain without the use of pharmacological agents, for they are seen infrequently. The role of suggestion in pain control is presented in Chapter 5.

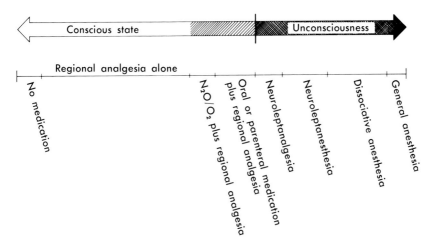

Fig. 2-1. The spectrum of pain control.

REGIONAL ANALGESIA

Without doubt, the vast majority of dental patients may undergo routine dental treatment with operative pain controlled through the use of regional analgesia alone. Its convenience, safety, and easy masterability make it one of dentistry's most valuable tools.

However, if it is to be used to fullest advantage, it must be well understood. Techniques for its administration are beyond the scope of this text and have been covered in another book, *Monheim's Local Anesthesia and Pain Control in Dental Practice*. It is suggested that the reader be thoroughly familiar with the technical aspects of regional analgesia administration. The importance of this means of pain control cannot be overstressed—whether it be used alone or in conjunction with other agents and techniques.

Note that the phrase *regional analgesia* was substituted for *local anesthesia* in the previous paragraph. This phrase was chosen because it more accurately describes the modality being discussed here.

By definition, *anesthesia* means the lack of all sensation. This is true whether the term is applied to regional or to general techniques. Similarly, the term *analgesia* refers to an inability to appreciate pain. However, in contrast to anesthesia, it must pertain only to regional techniques, since total general analgesia is an impossibility. With the drugs currently available it is impossible for a patient to be analgetic (free of all induced pain) and conscious at the same time.

The phrase *regional analgesia* requires some discussion if the concept of a spectrum of pain control is to be understood.

It is well known by all those who deal with pain control that when a local anesthetic solution is applied to a nerve trunk the fibers within that trunk are narcotized in a particular order. Those fibers transmitting pain are narcotized first, and fibers conducting temperature, touch, proprioception, and motor impulses follow in that order.

Generally speaking, the dentist desires and secures a blockade of only those nerve fibers capable of conducting the sensations that are interpreted as pain. Hence, *regional analgesia* rather than *local anesthesia* is produced. Patients may be able to feel pressure, touch, etc. while unable to appreciate painful stimuli.

As described in Chapter 1, the phenomenon of pain perception is quite similar from patient to patient and is the same in all patients from day to day. This aspect of pain is easily controlled with those drugs capable of interrupting the flow of painful impulses from the peripheral to the central nervous system.

On the other hand, pain reaction varies quite markedly and is influenced by numerous extraneous factors: emotional makeup, past experience, and the like.

It is conceivable, then, that a dental patient possessing satisfactory *regional analgesia* might subconsciously misinterpret other modalities (pressure, touch, etc.) as being painful during dental treatment. In other words, it may be extremely difficult to control pain with the use of regional analgesia alone in those patients who, owing to fear of dental treatment or recollection of a previously unpleasant dental experience, possess an altered pain reaction threshold. Therefore it becomes crucial that the practitioner be acutely aware of controlling both the pain perception and the pain reaction processes.

As a general rule, regional analgesia is not difficult to secure. A variety of pharmacological agents are available, the nerves in question are readily accessible, and techniques necessary are easily mastered. Once again, the importance of this aspect of pain control must be stressed.

The roles of fear, apprehension, emotional makeup, and past experience not only are significant in the realization of operative pain but also determine the patient's ability to psychologically cope with dental treatment (Chapter 4). Many patients realize the importance of routine dental care yet fail to seek treatment, out of fear of anticipated pain. Others do seek care but because of psychological conflicts are poor dental patients. They habitually break or are late for appointments, do not tolerate dental procedures well, chronically complain of minor discomforts, move incessantly during treatment, and generally make the day unpleasant for both themselves and the practitioner.

CONSCIOUS-SEDATION—AN ALTERNATIVE TO GENERAL ANESTHESIA

Before a discussion of this segment of the pain control spectrum can be undertaken, a definition of the word *conscious* is in order. The definition must be thoroughly understood, since it embodies the entire philosophy of conscious-sedation: *A patient is said to be conscious if he is capable of rational* *response to command and has all protective reflexes intact including the ability to clear and maintain his airway in a patent state.**

If conscious-sedation is to be employed, *all aspects* of the definition of conscious must be satisfied *at all times*. If any one aspect is violated for even a brief period, the patient is no longer in a conscious state. Rather, he has been placed in a life-threatening situation that is extremely hazardous, especially if the dentist lacks sufficient training, experience, equipment, and personnel to manage the situation.

On the other hand, if all criteria included in the definition are met at all times, the patient is in a comfortable, relaxed, and safe state that is well within the realm of general dental practice. The techniques of conscious-sedation are easily mastered and should be as much a part of dental practice as the administration of regional analgesia. The patient who is under the influence of conscious-sedation is in a well-controlled environment in which his ability to tolerate the stresses of dental treatment is greatly enhanced. The poorer the patient's physical and psychological condition, the greater the indication for conscious-sedation, as is elaborated in Chapter 3.

Objectives of conscious-sedation

Anyone who is to employ conscious-sedation successfully must realize and understand the objectives of the technique. When the dentist has a thorough understanding of the objectives in mind, the bounds of conscious-sedation are practically limitless. Without such understanding, it is fraught with dangers. *Understanding* is the by-word in conscious-sedation.

1. *The patient's mood must be altered.* Alteration of the patient's mood is the primary objective of conscious-sedation regardless of the technique or pharmacological agents employed. By appropriate alteration of the patient's mood two primary benefits are gained. First, the patient's pain reaction is altered. As previously discussed, such factors as fear and apprehension may alter the pain reaction to such an extent that nonpainful stimuli (for example, touch or pressure) may subconsciously be misinterpreted as pain. If fear and apprehension are eliminated and the patient is in a calmed, sedated, or euphoric state, he no longer misconstrues these sensations as being painful. In effect, the dentist is better able to control operative pain.

Second, after alteration of the patient's mood a procedure—namely, dental treatment—that was previously psychologically disturbing and not well accepted will be accepted willingly. The psychological conflict having been removed, he now becomes an eager dental patient. No longer do fears of unpleasant experiences in the dental office cause him to seek dental treatment and then break the appointment at the last minute. No longer does he force himself to keep the appointment but then psychologically reject treatment by

---

*From a definition by the American Dental Society of Anesthesiology, Inc.

being an uncooperative patient. Instead, having had his mood altered, he becomes the docile patient a dentist looks forward to treating.

2. *The patient must remain conscious.* When conscious-sedation is used, the patient must remain conscious *at all times.* He must respond rationally to verbal commands. This single entity is the best indicator of the state of consciousness. If the patient is incapable of appropriately responding to verbal commands after having been administered a sedative-type drug, the dentist must assume him to have been rendered unconscious. With the production of unconsciousness come certain deviations in physiological function, which may produce serious sequelae if not properly managed.

This is not to say that there may not be some alteration in state of awareness or that responses may not be sluggish. In fact, the usual result is that the patient may have slurred speech or may respond to commands more slowly than usual. Nevertheless, responses to command will be rational and appropriate.

3. *The patient must be cooperative.* Certainly, one of the main objectives must be to gain the cooperation of the patient. The individual who was previously fearful and uncooperative must be administered the proper drug or drugs in dosages sufficient to allay fear and apprehension and render him cooperative through alteration of his mood. Patient cooperation is one of the greatest advantages the *dentist* has to gain. The application of regional analgesia is facilitated, allowing the operator to better control operative pain. When this patient's pain is adequately controlled and his mood altered, he becomes a nearly ideal dental patient. Sitting comfortably still and in a cooperative mood, the patient allows the practitioner to perform his service in an unhurried yet efficient manner. As a result, both patient and dentist benefit. A greater amount of work can be accomplished in less than usual time. The patient benefits by having to make fewer trips to the dental office, while the dentist benefits by a greater productivity per time spent at the chair.

4. *All protective reflexes must remain intact and active.* The safety of conscious-sedative techniques is based on the fact that all protective reflexes remain active throughout the course of the sedative experience. This means that the patient's normal physiological parameters will continue to function properly *at all times.* The ability to cough and clear the airway remains active. The possibility of airway obstruction, from either foreign material or soft tissue, is no more possible in the patient under conscious-sedation than it is in the totally unmedicated patient.

Respiratory system reflexes remain active and intact. Deviations from normal in this system are not likely to occur. The patient will breathe normally and occasionally sigh as in the unmedicated state, thereby precluding entirely the possibility of hypoxia or hypercapnia.

Cardiovascular system reflexes will operate normally also. Under the influence of conscious-sedation a patient is not likely to become either hypotensive or hypertensive. Similarly, bradycardia and tachycardia will not occur, since homeostatic mechanisms are not interfered with.

Just as the ability to respond rationally to verbal command is the best indicator as to the state of consciousness, it is also assurance that all protective reflexes are operating to maintain vital functions within normal limits.

5. *Vital signs must remain stable and within normal limits.* It follows logically that if (a) the patient remains conscious and (b) all protective reflexes remain intact and active the vital signs will remain stable and within normal limits in the patient under conscious-sedation. This is not to say that vital signs will remain at preoperative levels throughout the appointment. Consider the apprehensive patient who, owing to his apprehension, presents for dental treatment with as elevated pulse rate and blood pressure. Once he has been seated in the dental chair and properly medicated, his vital signs usually decrease in value to fall within normal limits—reflecting the fact that apprehension, which was responsible for their elevation, has been eliminated.

Throughout the appointment there will be only mild deviations in vital signs, such as occur in all individuals. Moreover, the deviations will not range outside that patient's normal limits; that is, no fall in blood pressure, pulse rate, or respiratory rate and depth below the normal for that patient will occur.

I have personally monitored or supervised the monitoring in over 20,000 cases of conscious-sedation in the past 15 years, and in no instance was a serious deviation in vital signs noted. Proper attention to drug selection, dose, route, and rate of administration will preclude almost entirely the possibility of a serious change in vital function, even in the most seriously ill individual.

6. *The patient's pain threshold should be elevated.* Many times it is desirable for the patient's pain threshold to be elevated at a central nervous system level even though adequate regional analgesia has been secured. Any time a practitioner is relying on regional techniques for the control of operative pain he should bear in mind the fact that pain has a psychological as well as a physical component. For this reason it is wise to introduce drugs that also aid in the control of pain by altering the pain reaction. Even those individuals who appear to be acceptable dental patients may recall past experiences or harbor mild fears and thereby stand to benefit from an elevation of the pain threshold. Most often the agents that elevate the pain threshold also produce euphoria and freedom from fear, which contributes greatly toward alteration of mood.

There is yet another factor that makes elevation of the pain threshold desirable. Frequently, during the course of dental treatment the patient will experience discomfort at a site some distance from the operative area. For example, inadvertent trauma to the temporomandibular joint by pressure required to remove a deeply impacted mandibular third molar might cause the patient some discomfort. If an agent that elevates the pain threshold is administered during use of the conscious-sedative technique, an otherwise annoying occurrence may go unnoticed.

7. *Amnesia may be present.* Depending on the drug, dose, route, rate of administration, and desirability, amnesia for certain events may be produced in the conscious patient. Amnesia may not be produced nor is it desirable in all cases. But with a careful selection and/or combination of pharmacological effects the conscious patient may be placed in a state in which certain events, such as the administration of regional analgesia, are either poorly recalled or not recalled at all.

Amnesia is not necessary or warranted in all patients but may be a welcome adjunct in selected cases. For those individuals whose fear of the armamentarium associated with the production of regional analgesia has been a deterrent to the seeking of dental care, amnesia may be advisable. In other cases it may be of only minimal benefit.

Careful attention to patient responses during the pretreatment evaluation (Chapter 3) should enable the dentist to select those patients who might tolerate the dental procedure best if a degree of amnesia is present.

The seven objectives of conscious-sedation must be well understood if this means of controlling pain and apprehension is to be used successfully. As mentioned, several objectives must be achieved at all times whereas others, although beneficial, need not be present in every instance.

However, if the ones that have been deemed absolutely necessary are fulfilled, the patient will be free of pain, fear, and apprehension. He will be more able to physically and psychologically tolerate the dental procedure, while the dentist will prosper from the advantages to be gained from working with a patient who is calmed and cooperative.

If the objectives set forth are achieved, additional benefits are to be gained by both the patient and the practitioner. Because of the inherent safety of the procedure, continual monitoring of vital signs such as pulse, respiration, and blood pressure is not required, as it is with unconscious techniques. The patient is merely evaluated periodically for his state of consciousness, comfort, and cooperation. If these three parameters are present to a suitable degree, it may be assumed that physiological parameters are within normal limits.

Once again, owing to their inherent safety, conscious-sedative techniques do not require a special person for administration, as do unconscious techniques. The dentist who administers the sedation may also be the dentist who performs the necessary dental treatment. This is in direct contrast to unconscious techniques, in which *under no circumstances* should the operating dentist also be the individual who administers or directs the administration of any drugs that render the patient unconscious. Although the legal responsibility for the administration of unconscious techniques may rest with the operating dentist, the technical responsibility for such administration must rest with another individual, one who is specifically trained in management of the unconscious patient—namely, a nurse anesthetist, another dentist, or a physician.

Selection of the appropriate conscious-sedative technique

Obviously, conscious-sedation may be produced by a variety of drugs, doses, and routes of administration. In each instance, however, it is accompanied by the use of regional analgesia for the control of operative pain.

The dentist is therefore confronted with the selection of the conscious-sedative technique best suited to his needs and the requirements of each patient. Although various drugs, doses, and routes of administration will be dealt with in subsequent chapters, let me say here that, within the spectrum of pain control, one must also be aware of the spectrum of techniques available. In other words, myriad drugs, drug combinations, dosages, and routes of administration exist; the practitioner has an infinite number of techniques, on a continuum, from which to choose.

The knowledgeable practitioner should not attempt to devise a conscious-sedative technique consisting of specific drugs, doses, rates, and intervals of administration and attempt to make "his technique" suit all patients. Rather, he should understand the concept of conscious-sedation and the objectives sought; he should become familiar with the pharmacology of categories of drugs, rather than specific drug entities; he should understand the advantages and disadvantages of specific routes of administration. Then he should be able to intelligently blend the components into a conscious-sedative technique that will fill the needs of both patient and doctor. The practitioner who employs a predetermined technique regardless of the patient's physical and psychological needs is demonstrating a lack of knowledge and understanding, which precludes one of the great advantages of conscious-sedation, flexibility!

Whereas a technique based on understanding is most likely to be successful, one based on a "recipe" or "cocktail" will frequently be less than satisfactory and, on occasion, hazardous.

Levels of awareness

That he may select the conscious-sedative technique best suited to a particular patient, the dentist must become aware of another concept relevant to sedation. I have arbitrarily termed this concept "level of awareness."

If I may digress for a moment and discuss general anesthesia, a parallel may be drawn that will clarify the "level of awareness" concept.

In 1920 Guedel described the signs and stages of ether anesthesia, in an attempt to relate the dose of the agent with the "depth" of anesthesia. He had been forced to study this correlation because his responsibilities during World War I were such that the shortage of anesthetists required a training of corpsmen of administer general anesthesia for battle casualties. In effect he summarized a series of signs that would be obvious to the relatively untrained individual and would serve as an indicator of proper dosage. If the dose administered was greater than necessary, the patient (literally, the anesthesia) was said to be "too deep." Conversely, if insufficient doses were administered, the patient was said to be "too light."

The signs and stages that Guedel set forth have been shown to be quite accurate—but for ether anesthesia only. His signs and stages are not applicable to any other agent. However, the idea of clear-cut signs and stages has stayed with us, as has the idea of *depth* of anesthesia.

A better understanding of the pharmacology of anesthetic agents has led to a realization that depth of anesthesia is relative to the degree of stimulation. For example, it is well known that pain is an effective narcotic antagonist. A dose that may be considered appropriate in the presence of pain may be an overdose in its absence. Similarly, a patient may appear to be deeply anesthetized in the absence of painful stimuli. Blood pressure, pulse rate, and respiratory functions may be well below satisfactory limits. However, when painful stimuli are applied, it soon becomes obvious that the patient is lightly rather than deeply narcotized.

A similar analogy may be drawn with conscious-sedative techniques. Assume, for example, that a given "level of awareness" within a patient is such that dental procedures may be carried out comfortably (Fig. 2-2). By far the majority of patients will arrive in the office in this state and will require no medication other than regional analgesia.

Some patients, on the other hand, will be mildly apprehensive and must be sedated to a level of awareness at which dental procedures will be comfortably tolerated. These mildly apprehensive patients may be satisfactorily managed with the use of mild pharmacological agents such as nitrous oxide, the weakest agent known for the production of conscious-sedation. The patient who is very

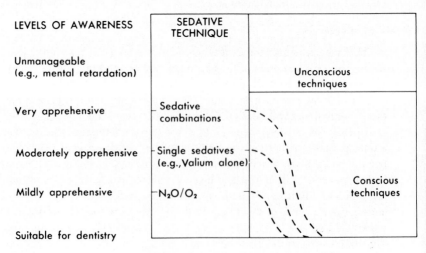

Fig. 2-2. Levels of awareness.

mildly apprehensive may be managed with very low doses of this weak agent, whereas one who is a bit more apprehensive may require greater doses.

Nitrous oxide, being a very weak agent, may not be sufficiently potent to manage a moderately apprehensive patient. Therefore a "ceiling effect" is produced. Some patients will require drugs more potent than nitrous oxide and oxygen if they are to be managed satisfactorily in the conscious state. To manage the more difficult patient the dentist may consider adding other agents, such as orally active drugs, to the inhalation of nitrous oxide and oxygen. For those patients exhibiting a modest degree of fear and apprehension, he may choose to control anxieties with single injectable drugs, which are even more potent. Patients who exhibit a great deal of fear and apprehension may require multiple-drug combinations if their "level of awareness" is to be lowered sufficiently for dentistry to be satisfactorily performed. Many patients will not only require more potent drugs but may also require a combination of drugs and routes of administration.

Just as the depth of general anesthesia is related to the degree of stimulation, the degree of conscious-sedation required is related to the level of awareness (or apprehension) that the patient presents. Mildly apprehensive patients may be managed with relatively weak agents. In contrast, those patients having a greater degree of apprehension will require more potent drugs, larger doses, or more sophisticated combinations. Clearly, there is not only a spectrum of pain control, containing a spectrum of techniques within it; there is also a mini-spectrum of drugs and doses within the techniques available.

Just as a "ceiling effect" was demonstrated for nitrous oxide and oxygen alone, a ceiling exists for all forms of conscious-sedation. It is not possible for all patients to be managed in the conscious state, with all the objectives set forth earlier being attained. For example, no amount of conscious-sedation will instill cooperativeness in a mentally handicapped individual. The patient must possess certain inherent behavioral and intellectual attributes that are indispensable if conscious-sedation is to be successful.

It is my belief, therefore, that certain individuals must be managed with the use of unconscious techniques, and their management must fall into the hands of individuals specifically trained in such procedures. However, it is also my belief that in far too many instances the patient is considered a candidate for an unconscious technique because neither the patient nor the operator realizes what may be accomplished in the conscious state. I believe that any *dental procedure* that can be accomplished in a dental office can be accomplished without resort to unconscious techniques. This, of course, assumes the patient to possess certain minimal and basic behavioral and intellectual attributes. General anesthesia must not be employed either as a convenience to the dentist or because the patient "wants to go to sleep." It is the practitioner's responsibility to educate the patient, as well as himself, to the advantages of conscious-sedation.

UNCONSCIOUS TECHNIQUES

So that the reader may be familiar with the principles, advantages, and pitfalls of unconscious techniques, a brief discussion of these areas will follow.

Once the patient is no longer in harmony with his surroundings (that is, he is no longer capable of rational response to command), he must be considered to be unconscious. With the production of unconsciousness come certain deviations in physiological function, which are definitely life threatening in the absence of someone trained in the management of the condition produced. A state of unconsciousness from which one cannot be aroused is certain to produce partial or complete airway obstruction that will ultimately result in hypoxia, hypercapnia, and the eventual death of the patient. In addition, many other reflexes are abolished or obtunded, frequently resulting in wide deviations in respiratory and cardiovascular system function. The patient loses the ability to clear his tracheobronchial tree; respiratory depression, with its attendant blood gas and the pH changes, occurs; and cardiovascular system function may deteriorate, as well.

When vital protective reflexes are lost or obtunded, a trained individual must be present to, essentially, *become* the reflex system of the patient. He must pay constant attention to and provide corrective measures for the changes that are certain to occur in vital functions that have been placed in a labile state. The argument that deviations from normal are not likely to occur in one who is only lightly anesthetized or is unconscious for only a brief period is a ludicrous statement that only serves to demonstrate the ignorance of anyone expounding such a philosophy. All unconscious techniques must be understood before use and must be treated with respect at all times.

Such constant attention to vital functions is required at all times that *one* individual who has been trained for at least a year in general anesthesia must constantly maintain a patent airway and monitor vital signs (pulse, respiration, blood pressure, etc.), while taking appropriate measures to safeguard the life and welfare of the patient.

Neuroleptanalgesia. Neuroleptanalgesia is a relative new technique, which employs narcotic analgetics up to 150 times as potent as morphine. Potent psychosedatives are also employed. The combination results in an intense analgetic and amnesic state in a patient quite calmed and detached from his surroundings. Respiratory and circulatory changes are frequent and require constant monitoring along with corrective and supportive measures when indicated. The patient may or may not be rendered unconscious.

Neuroleptanesthesia. A combination of neuroleptanalgesia plus inhalation of nitrous oxide and oxygen results in the production of neuroleptanesthesia. In this case the patient is definitely rendered unconscious. Although discontinuance of nitrous oxide and oxygen results in a prompt return to consciousness, the patient's vital reflexes may remain severely obtunded for extended periods of time and require constant supervision.

Dissociative anesthesia. The only drug presently available for the production of dissociative anesthesia is ketamine hydrochloride (Ketalar, Ketaject). Dissociative anesthesia is characterized by unconsciousness, amnesia, and intensive analgesia coupled with a cataleptic appearance. Cardiovascular and respiratory system functions are remarkably stable, and protective reflexes remain normal or somewhat hyperreactive. On occasion, hyperreactive reflexes may result in troublesome tongue movements, producing difficult conditions for intraoral procedures. Accentuation of airway reflexes occasionally leads to laryngospasm in which the use of a neuromuscular blocking agent is required for control.

Approximately 15% of adult patients will experience vivid and bizarre dreams while under the influence of dissociative anesthesia. This may result from the fact that ketamine selectively interrupts association pathways of the brain before producing somesthetic blockade. It may selectively depress the thalamoneocortical system before obtunding the more ancient cerebral centers and pathways (reticular-activating and limbic systems).

General anesthesia. The state of general anesthesia lies at the opposite end of the spectrum from that in which the patient is in the alert, conscious, unmedicated state. The patient under general anesthesia is unconscious, his pain eliminated through depression of higher nervous system centers, and has many protective reflexes obtunded. He is literally at the mercy of the anesthetist and owes his very life to the conscientious attention of the individual who is responsible for having rendered him totally inappreciative of all sensation.

As with any unconscious technique, vital functions must be monitored continually by the *one* individual responsible for the life and welfare of the patient. It is totally inconceivable that anyone can successfully rationalize his ability to administer or supervise the administration of an unconscious technique by an untrained individual while simultaneously performing dental treatment.

CONSCIOUS VERSUS UNCONSCIOUS TECHNIQUES

Table 1 contrasts the primary differences between conscious and unconscious techniques. Many aspects contained in the table have been discussed but deserve further attention at this time.

In addition, the incidence of operative and postoperative complications with conscious-sedation is extremely low compared to that with unconscious techniques. A certain amount of trauma is generally associated with even the most careful administration of unconscious techniques, which is not present when conscious techniques are employed. Pressures required for such procedures as maintenance of the airway or insertion of a mouth prop or an endotracheal tube frequently result in annoying if not serious postoperative problems.

Convenience to the patient as well as the dentist is afforded by conscious-

Table 1. Conscious versus unconscious techniques

Conscious	Unconscious
Mood altered	Patient unconscious
Patient conscious	Patient unconscious
Patient cooperative	No patient cooperation
Protective reflexes active and intact	Protective reflexes obtunded
	Airway may become obstructed
	Respiratory—hypoxia or hypercapnia
	Cardiovascular—hypotension or hypertension; bradycardia or tachycardia
Vital signs stable	Vital signs labile
Analgesia may be present	Pain eliminated centrally
Regional analgesia usually required	Regional analgesia not required
Amnesia may be present	Amnesia always present
Operating dentist may perform sedation	Operating dentist must *not* act also as anesthetist
Minimum amount of equipment required	Special equipment necessary
No additional personnel required	Additional trained personnel required
	Nurse anesthetist
	Dentist anesthetist
	Physician anesthetist
	Recovery room personnel
Prolonged detainment in recovery room not required	Detainment in recovery area necessary
Some patients (having N_2O/O_2 only) may be discharged unescorted	All patients must be escorted home
Risk of complications very low	Risk of complications high
Postoperative complications infrequent	Postoperative complications not infrequent
Extremely difficult or mentally handicapped patient cannot always be managed	May be only method by which extremely difficult or mentally handicapped patient can be managed
Preoperative laboratory tests not required	Preoperative laboratory tests required
Food intake restricted	Food intake forbidden for 6 to 8 hours
Convenient in an office	Inconvenient in an office
Excellent choice for poor-risk patient in dental office	Not indicated for poor-risk patient in dental office

sedation. The patient need not undergo special laboratory tests, need not fast for an extended period prior to the appointment, and need not be unduly detained after the procedure. In those instances in which conscious-sedation has been achieved with the use of nitrous oxide alone with oxygen, he need not be escorted from the office. As a general rule the poor-risk patient may safely and comfortably undergo dental treatment in the office with the aid of conscious-sedation. The same patient will require hospitalization with its associated inconvenience and cost if unconscious techniques must be employed.

Once again I must state this as my firm opinion. With few exceptions, any *dental procedure* that can be performed in a dental office can be satisfactorily managed with a combination of regional analgesia plus conscious-sedation.

If this premise is accepted, the indications for unconscious techniques will decline rapidly. The fearful, apprehensive patient will undergo dental treatment in a comfortable state in the dental office. Once patients realize that the dentist is considerate and is capable of managing their problems appropriately and efficiently, the profession will be in a position to more effectively deliver dental health care. Patients will be appreciative of the kind and thoughtful care they receive.

Chapter 3

PREOPERATIVE PATIENT EVALUATION

Before he is given any dental treatment, each prospective patient must undergo a thorough history and physical evaluation. This is an extremely valuable procedure from which much useful information may be gained. Not only does it, as a part of the dentist's records, become a document of legal importance; it also allows the dentist to determine the patient's physical and psychological ability to tolerate the dental procedure, and thus it enables the practitioner to select those patients who may benefit from the use of conscious-sedation. In addition it plays a major role in the management and prevention of office emergencies.

Today the importance of an adequate pretreatment evaluation is greater than ever before. Because of the advances in medical care many patients who previously might have succumbed in their illness, or at best been confined to their beds or homes, are now active, contributing members of our society. Their very lives are being sustained through pharmacodynamic mechanisms. As a result, they are not only leading relatively normal lives; they are also seeking dental treatment as a part of their regular routine.

The dentist therefore bears the responsibility not only for rendering competent dental service but also for understanding each patient's general physical and psychological condition so that needed dental treatment may be completed without exaggerating any existing but therapeutically compensated pathology.

It must be borne in mind that the dentist is securing pertinent information in an effort to evaluate the dental situation—not to diagnose or to treat the patient for any medical problem. The evaluation should enable the dentist to determine *how* the patient should be treated and not *who* should be treated. The practitioner no longer has the luxury of treating only healthy patients; it is his obligation to treat all patients who seek dental care. The evaluation will enable the dentist to determine how each individual should be managed and what precautions, if any, must be taken to safeguard the life and welfare of the patient.

The evaluation need not be unduly time-consuming or cumbersome. However, to proceed without any evaluation whatsoever is unwarranted. All negative as well as positive findings must be made a part of the patient's permanent record and be readily available for future reference. The information must also be periodically updated so that the dentist will be aware of all changes in the patient's condition that may be relevant to the case.

Generally speaking, the pretreatment evaluation may be considered valid if it was performed within 6 months of dental treatment. This does not mean that the entire evaluation page need be rewritten. Rather, only those changes that have taken place need be noted. Certainly, all new positive finding should be pursued to their fullest, to determine the extent to which dental treatment must be altered.

Adverse circumstances have taught many a dentist that not all patients are good candidates for dental service, from either a physical or a psychological standpoint, when managed indiscriminately. When the practitioner has determined the true condition of the patient by means of an adequate pretreatment evaluation, he is better able to plan his treatment, schedule appointments, select the conscious-sedative technique best suited to his and the patient's needs, and deliver dental care in a relaxed and efficient manner.

The pretreatment evaluation not only enables the dentist to determine the patient's ability to withstand the stress of dental treatment but also enables him to identify the need for conscious-sedation, the sedative technique required, and the drugs that may be employed. When these factors are coupled with pertinent dental findings, the dentist is able to formulate a treatment plan—one designed with safety, comfort, productivity, and efficiency in mind.

Preliminary information concerning the patient such as name, age, sex, height, weight, and occupation may be secured by an office assistant rather than the dentist. The remaining information necessary to complete the evaluation should be obtained by the dentist himself in the first few minutes of the initial appointment. The examiner should develop a somewhat standardized procedure for the history to assure its completeness and efficiency. The taking of a good history necessitates that the examiner ask the questions and listen attentively to the answers. It is a serious error and an ill-advised shortcut to give the patient a list of questions and permit him to circle a "yes" or "no" answer.

The fundamentals involved in history taking are to ask clear, concise questions, to listen attentively, to observe, and to integrate. The questions should not be confusing to the patient, and they should be asked in a manner that will elicit the most useful information. The patient should not be unduly cut short when answering. Listening to and sifting the answers is an art, as is asking the questions. A good listener will derive much more information from verbal replies than is obtainable from written answers. Many times the *manner* in which the question is answered will indicate that the question was not understood or will supply more information than the answer that is given.

The dentist should always remember that he is securing pertinent information to evaluate and not to diagnose or treat the patient for any medical problem.

On the first visit the dentist must also perform a brief physical examination, including a determination of blood pressure and the pulse rate, rhythm, and character. All findings should be entered into the patient's permanent record. Comments concerning the findings should not be made to the patient.

The dentist should depend on his pretreatment evaluation to determine each of the following.

PRE-TREATMENT MEDICAL EVALUATION

DATE

NAME - LAST. FIRST. MIDDLE	MARITAL STAT.	AGE	DATE OF BIRTH MO. DAY YR.	SEX	HT.	WT

ADDRESS	PHONE	OCCUPATION	RACIAL GROUP

FAMILY PHYSICIAN - NAME.   ADDRESS.   PHONE NO.

A GENERAL
1. What is your general state of health?
2. Are you now or have you recently been under a physician s care?_____ Reason
3. Are you now taking or within the past 6 months have you taken any drugs or medications?
   Names: _____ Reason:
4. Have you ever had a serious illness or operation?_____ Describe:
5. Do you have any allergies?_____To what:
6. Have you ever had a reaction to a local anesthetic, antibiotic, or other drug?
   Describe:
7. Are you pregnant?_____Month?_____Number pregnancy?
8. Have you ever had hepatitis or been jaundiced?
9. Have you ever had veneral disease? (Gonorrhea or Syphilis)

B. CARDIOVASCULAR — RESPIRATORY
1. Are you able to perform your daily duties without stress or strain?
2. Are your activities limited for any reason?
3. Have you ever had any chest pains?
4. Have you ever had any shortness of breath?
5. Do you have a cough or wheeze?
6. Have you ever coughed up blood?
7. Do you ever have dizzy spells?
8. Can you lie flat when lying down or sleeping?
9. Do your ankles swell?_____When?
10. Have you ever been aware of a rapid heart beat or palpitations?
11. Have you ever had rheumatic fever?
12. Have you ever been told you had a heart murmur, heart trouble, or lung trouble?
13. Do you have frequent colds, sore throats or sinus trouble?
14. Have you ever had night sweats?_____When?

C. HEMATOPOIETIC
1. Have you ever had prolonged bleeding following a cut, tooth extraction, or other injury?
2. Have you ever had x-ray treatments or irradiation?_____ When?_____ Why?
3. Have you ever been told you were anemic?
4. Do you bruise easily?
5. Do you experience nose bleeds?
6. Do you have frequent infections?
7. Have you ever had a blood transfusion?_____Why?

D. NERVOUS SYSTEM
1. Have you ever had a convulsion or seizure?
2. Are you troubled by frequent headaches?
3. Are you frequently unduly apprehensive, fearful, or nervous?
4. Do you ever experience any pains, numbness or tingling anywhere?
5. Have you ever consulted a psychiatrist?

E. METABOLIC — ENDOCRINE
1. Have you had any recent gain or loss of weight?_____ Pounds?
2. Do you have a good appetite?
3. Does heat or warm rooms make you uncomfortable?
4. Do your hands sweat excessively?
5. Are you a diabetic?_____ How long?_____ Treatment?
6. Are you easily fatigued?

1. Patient's general physical condition
2. Patient's ability to physically and psychologically tolerate the stress of the dental procedure
3. Need for medical consultation
4. Need for conscious-sedation
5. Conscious-sedative technique and degree of sedation required
6. Time to be allotted for the procedure
7. Choice of drugs (including regional analgetic and vasoconstrictor agents)

PRE-TREATMENT MEDICAL EVALUATION

F. GENITOURINARY
1. Do you void frequently?
2. Do you have to get up at night to void?
3. Do you have any difficulty in voiding?
4. Have you ever had blood in your urine?
5. Have you ever been told you had kidney trouble?

G. SOCIAL & PERSONAL
1. Is there any history of tuberculosis, diabetes, or bleeding in your family?
2. Do you smoke? _____ What? _____ How much?
3. Do you drink? _____ How much?
4. Are your wife and children in good health?

PHYSICAL EXAMINATION

BLOOD PRESSURE	PULSE RATE	VOLUME	RHYTHM	TEMPERATURE	RESPIRATIONS	DEPTH	CHARACTER
	/MIN.				/MIN.		

INDICATE WHETHER FINDINGS ARE POSITIVE (+) OR NEGATIVE (—)

SKIN - _____ JAUNDICE _____ PALLOR _____ PETECHIAE _____ ECCHYMOSIS

_____ CYNOSIS _____ RASH _____ OTHER

HEAD - _____ DEFORMITY _____ SWELLING _____ OTHER

EYES - _____ JAUNDICE _____ EXOPHTHALMOS _____ MOVEMENT

_____ REDNESS _____ OTHER

HANDS - _____ CLUBBING _____ PIGMENTATION _____ TREMOR _____ TEMP.

_____ OTHER

NECK - _____ LYMPH NODES _____ THYROID _____ VEINS _____ OTHER

LEGS - _____ EDEMA _____ ULCERS _____ CYANOSIS _____ OTHER

ANY OTHER PHYSICAL DEFECTS

DESCRIBE ANY ABNORMALTY OR POSITIVE FINDING

The pretreatment evaluation should be so well planned and organized that all necessary information can be secured with a minimum of time and effort on the part of the office personnel. It should cause little or no concern to the patient, particularly when he is informed that it is a routine procedure.

A sheet or card should be printed with all necessary questions as an aid in conducting a uniform evaluation. An example of such a form is shown on pp. 26 and 27.

In addition to the general needs mentioned above, specific areas of concern to the dentist should include the following;

1. Status of the patient's cardiovascular and respiratory systems
2. Nervous system disorders
3. Metabolic deficiencies
4. Endocrine imbalances
5. Allergic manifestations
6. Medications the patient may be taking
7. Hematologic pathologies
8. Iatrogenic conditions
9. Psychological or emotional instability

CARDIOVASCULAR STATUS

Generally the status of the cardiovascular system will be of prime importance to the dentist, since its pathological disturbances may produce alarming results. Practically all patients whose cardiovascular systems are sufficiently impaired to cause concern are under the care of a physician and take medication for their condition. There are many ambulatory patients whose cardiovascular mechanisms are such that they are unable to tolerate the stress of dental treatment unless certain precautions are taken. It has been stated that 10 to 14 million people are known to have some form of heart disease, and it is probable that an equal number have undiagnosed cardiovascular disease.

The cardiovascular conditions most likely to be of concern to the dentist may be divided into two groups: congenital heart disease and acquired heart disease.

Congenital heart disease

Congenital heart disease is the result of developmental defects of the heart and/or major blood vessels. When the defect is profound, the prognosis is poor and death usually occurs early. However, some persons with unrepaired, marked heart defects may survive long enough (two decades) to require dental treatment.

As a general rule these patients can be recognized by their general retardation in growth and maturation. In addition the skin, lips, and nailbeds may be cyanotic or pale, and often the fingers are clubbed. Activity is usually reduced in direct proportion to the severity of the condition. This means that they have a poor exercise tolerance and get out of breath easily.

These individuals may not be able to tolerate the stresses associated with long or trying dental procedures, particularly if they are fearful individuals. Their appointments should be kept to a minimum length and must be free of pain. Conscious-sedation may be employed to advantage, but care must be taken to be sure that heavy sedation is avoided. Generally, the elimination of fear and apprehension will allow them to better tolerate the dental procedure.

Patients who have had corrective surgery for congenital cardiovascular defects will have a better exercise tolerance than those with defects unrepaired. They, too, will fare better if the appointment is pain-free and anxiety-free and the duration is kept to a minimum.

Patients falling into this category, whether they present repaired or unrepaired defects, should be medicated prophylactically with antibiotics prior to surgical procedures, as are the patients with a history of rheumatic fever. These individuals also run a substantial risk of contracting postoperative subacute bacterial endocarditis.

Acquired heart disease

Acquired heart disease, with the exception of rheumatic heart disease, is most prevalent after 40 years of age. The dentist must be cognizant of the somewhat common occurrence of these conditions and of the possibility that patients with such conditions may appear in the dental office for treatment.

Acquired heart disease can be classified as follows:
1. Rheumatic heart disease
2. Atherosclerotic heart disease
   a. Angina pectoris   b. Coronary artery disease
3. Hypertension
4. Hypotension
5. Pending congestive heart failure
6. Conductive system defects

Rheumatic heart disease

Rheumatic heart disease is primarily a disease of childhood and early adolescence, although many young and middle-aged adults are affected by its results. Since statistics conservatively estimate that there are more than a million cases of rheumatic heart disease in the United States, the dentist must take an adequate case history to discover, if at all possible, the presence of this condition in any patient.

Even though the disease affects the myocardium and pericardium, it is endocardial involvement that produces the disability and resultant interference with valvular function. Most frequently, the mitral valve is involved.

Shortness of breath and intermittent fevers coupled with an elevated pulse rate in a young individual, even one with a negative history, should arouse the dentist's suspicion of rheumatic heart disease and indicate the need for consultation with a physician.

Patients relating a history of rheumatic fever should be given an antibiotic prior to surgery, to prevent development of subacute bacterial endocarditis. Those patients with a history of rheumatic fever who have also a history of a poor exercise tolerance may be considered as candidates for regional analgesia plus conscious-sedation.

The presence of a residual heart murmur, per se, need not indicate a need for conscious-sedation if emotional stability and a good exercise tolerance are present.

Atherosclerotic heart disease

Atherosclerotic heart disease, or coronary artery disease, is responsible for both angina pectoris and coronary thrombosis and accounts for about 25% of all heart disease in the United States.

Angina pectoris. The primary symptom of angina pectoris is the occurrence of sudden episodes of substernal pain that radiates down the left arm and to the left angle of the mandible. While it is known that atherosclerosis is an underlying factor, the immediate cause is unknown. The most widely held opinion is that a reduction of blood flow causes a temporary spasm of the coronary arteries. A more recent theory states that catecholamine release, resulting from sympathetic nervous system stimulation, increases the oxygen consumption of the myocardium, producing hypoxia of the myocardium with resultant pain.

Over half of the patients who are known to have coronary artery disease do not suffer anginal pains, although arteriosclerotic artery disease is an underlying factor. It is most common in men over 50 years of age, especially when it is associated with, for example, diabetes mellitus, Bueger's disease, polycythemia, severe anemia, or hyperthyroidism.

The following triad of symptoms is associated with angina pectoris: (1) the location and radiating nature of the pain, (2) the short duration of the attack, and (3) the immediate causative factors.

Most frequently an attack will be brought on by physical exertion, emotional episodes, or sudden exposure to cold environmental temperature. Attacks often occur after large meals.

It is of particular interest to the dentist to note that the pain may be most noticeable in the lower teeth or jaw, to the extent that the patient may seek dental treatment for the paroxysmal attacks of pain.

From the dentist's point of view the anginal patient can usually be recognized from the history. The pain is brought on by characteristic events, is of short duration, and subsides with rest. The pain is usually sharp and not viselike or excruciating. Although death may occur immediately following an attack of angina pectoris, it usually does not unless there is an associated coronary artery thrombosis.

Patients giving a history of angina pectoris will usually be taking medication such as a long-acting coronary vasodilator and will carry a short-acting agent such as nitroglycerin to alleviate sporadic attacks that may occur. The dentist must encourage the patient to take prescribed medications as directed. In addition, since physically as well as emotionally trying episodes may trigger attacks, the patient should reap the benefits of conscious-sedation and adequate regional analgesia for dental treatment.

Coronary artery disease. Patients who suffer from coronary artery disease are subject to coronary thrombosis or "heart attacks." History of a previous "coronary" or "heart attack" is ready evidence of coronary artery disease. The dentist must determine how long a time has elapsed since the last attack, what activities the patient is permitted, and what medication, if any, the patient is taking.

Coronary artery disease usually becomes evident in patients who are in their fourth, fifth, and sixth decades of life. Its only initial symptom may be attacks of paroxysmal dyspnea. A decided change in a person's ability to withstand physical exertion should be significant to the history taker. The time lapse since any previous attack is important, since a patient who has had no symptoms for over 2 years and is carrying out routine duties without stress or strain should be considered normal for his age group.

The use of vasoconstrictors in the regional analgetic agent is *not* contraindicated in patients with atherosclerotic heart disease. However, the concentration should be kept at 1:100,000 (0.01 mg./ml.), or lower, and the total dosage be restricted to 0.1 mg. or less.

It is worthwhile to note that attacks of angina pectoris or coronary artery occlusion frequently occur when large meals are coupled with a stressful or emotional situation. Patients who are subject to angina pectoris or who have coronary artery disease should be advised to eat lightly, if at all, immediately preceding a dental appointment. These patients should be spared any discomfort during dental appointments by the use of regional analgesia plus conscious-sedation. Long, tiring appointments should be avoided.

Hypertension

Blood pressure is the sum of cardiac output, blood volume, blood viscosity, and vessel elasticity and can be affected by any one of these factors. The blood pressure can be misleading, and at times it tells little about the actual state of the circulation. Thus wide variations in blood pressure occur normally.

However, a persistently high blood pressure (hypertension), which has been arbitrarily defined as one greater that 150/90, may lead to hypertensive heart disease and to eventual heart failure. It should be understood that hypertension is not a disease but a symptom. The normal systolic pressure for adults is from 90 to 130 mm. Hg and the diastolic pressure from 60 to 80 mm. Hg. Contrary to popular belief, the values of normal pressures attained during adolescence are maintained throughout life. It is not normal for pressures to increase with age. Thus the old guideline of "100 plus your age" as a normal for systolic pressure is not valid in the middle and older age groups.

Hypertension is quite common among older individuals. About 75% of all deaths occurring in persons over the age of 50 result from or are related to hypertension. The earliest form of hypertension is termed "labile hypertension." Here the resting blood pressure is only occasionally greater than 150/90. Between times at which the blood pressure is elevated come periods when it is within normal limits. If the abnormality is left unchecked, the most common form of hypertension, essential, benign, or more properly, idiopathic hypertension, will ensue. Idiopathic hypertension may produce very few symptoms, and the patient may exhibit no signs of discomfort whatsoever. The dentist, through routine pretreatment evaluations, may be the first member of the health team to detect hypertension. Other patients with these types of hypertension will present for routine dental treatment. They may be under the care of a physician and may be taking a variety of antihypertensive medications. It is imperative that the dentist familiarize himself with the pharmacology and actions of these drugs prior to undertaking dental treatment.

Malignant hypertension, in contrast to the other types, presents definite symptoms such as headache, dizziness, and occasional impairment of vision. Two of its earliest signs may be breathlessness after exertion and occasional nosebleeds. The medical history plus the blood pressure will most likely show the presence of malignant hypertension. In such cases the patients' blood pressure may be sustained at levels well above 180/100 and will not respond well to antihypertensive medications.

Those patients with moderate hypertension who exhibit no other symptoms may be treated as normal in every respect. However, in patients who relate symptoms of a poor exercise tolerance it is most advisable to employ a conscious-sedative technique coupled with regional analgesia.

As in patients who present with atherosclerotic heart disease, a vasoconstrictor may be employed along with the analgetic agent, but its dosage should be kept to a minimum.

Hypotension

Arterial hypotension is, as a rule, no cause for concern to the dentist. A systolic pressure of 90 or below with a diastolic pressure of 60 or below is arbitrarily defined as hypotension. Many persons with blood pressures in these ranges are without distress and function normally. Those normally hypotensive patients who have no other apparent physiological deviation are in satisfactory condition for any dental procedure. Those patients exhibiting additional symptoms such as dizziness or weakness should be referred to a physician for consultation prior to elective dental procedures.

Pending congestive heart failure

Patients who are in borderline congestive heart failure are among the most hazardous the dentist will be called on to treat in his office. A large number of such patients are ambulatory and are receiving treatment from a physician. These patients are thus potential appointees in the dental office.

A good history should forewarn the dentist if a patient shows pending congestive heart failure. In practically all such cases the patient is under the care of a physician and will make this fact known. Usually he is taking medication, most likely a cardiac glycoside, and his activities are restricted because of poor exercise tolerance. In many cases the large veins of the neck will be prominent and a nonproductive cough will be present. Ankle edema may be observed, especially in late afternoon, and the patient may have orthopnea (difficulty in breathing when lying flat). Several pillows may be required for sleeping, so that he can breathe easily. Such a patient should be treated with caution, to avoid a tachycardia that might exaggerate the condition already existing. Use of preoperative and operative conscious-sedation plus adequate regional analgesia is paramount in the management of any patient having these symptoms or history. He must not be exposed to the stress and strain of a poorly managed dental office visit.

It would be of particular benefit to closely and frequently observe the pulse rate of such a patient during dental procedures. The practitioner can very easily and inconspicuously palpate the pulse in the head and neck area without causing the patient undue concern. Should a marked increase in pulse rate occur, a rest period may be required. The need for the judicious use of conscious-sedation in these patients cannot be overstressed.

Chronic valvular heart disease

Chronic valvular heart disease refers to any permanent organic deformity of one or more of the cardiac valves. The valves may become stenotic, insufficient, or both. In all cases of "chronic valvular heart disease" the causative condition has become chronic or quiescent. Rheumatic fever is the underlying cause of the majority of valvular lesions that exist today, although other causes may be congenital anomalies, syphilis, healed bacterial endocarditis, atherosclerosis, and trauma.

Valvular heart disease is named for the valve affected and will thus be classified as in the following discussion.

Mitral valvular disease. Mitral valvular disease is practically always caused by rheumatic heart disease and is by far the most common form of chronic valvular disorder. This condition usually produces its most severe effects in adults who are young or of early middle age.

Aortic valvular disease. Aortic valvular disease occurs much less frequently than does mitral valvular disease. When it does occur, it is mostly in men over 50 years of age. The condition thus develops slowly and may, for a time, be well compensated. Later, however, anginal pain may appear and be quite severe.

Pulmonic valvular disease. Pulmonic valvular disease is relatively rare and is usually congenital in origin. Unless other diseases complicate the condition, the patient in such cases may lead a normal, moderately active life. When combined with other lesions, the condition can be extremely debilitating.

Tricuspid valvular disease. Tricuspid valvular disease rarely occurs as a separate entity; it is usually associated with lesions of the mitral valve and thus is almost invariably of rheumatic origin.

$$\bullet \quad \bullet \quad \bullet$$

The fact that practically all valvular lesions of any significance are of rheumatic or sclerotic origin is of importance to the dentist. The accompanying murmurs may or may not be important, depending on the time of their occurrence and the degree of compensation. A systolic murmur (one heard during contraction of the ventricles) may not always be indicative of valvular damage. However, a diastolic murmur (one heard during relaxation of the ventricles) is almost always indicative of cardiac valvular damage.

Practically all patients who have valvular heart disease either are or have been under the care of a physician. Many may have had one or more valves surgically repaired or replaced with artificial appliances. The dentist must question each patient regarding medications he may be taking and must determine the scope of that patient's daily activities and his ability to carry them out. Any patient who is able to perform an average load of daily activities, regardless of the presence of murmur, should present no problem during routine dental treatment.

The patient with a limited exercise tolerance, however, will fare better with the use of conscious-sedation plus regional analgesia obtained through an agent that includes a vasoconstrictor.

Cardiac arrhythmias

The normal heart beats with a regular rhythm produced by a stimulus originating in the sinoatrial node. The impulse spreads in a radial fashion over the atria to the atrioventricular (also called auriculoventricular) node, which lies posteriorly in the auriculoventricular septum. The impulse then spreads forward to the interauricular septum and continues into the ventricles over the bundle of His. This bundle divides into a right and a left branch at the superior end of the interventricular septum. The two branches (right and left) continue downward on either side of the interventricular septum and finally subdivide into the Purkinje fibers, which spread throughout the ventricles. Any interference with the initiating impulse at the sinoatrial node or with its spread throughout the conductive system will produce an arrhythmia.

The normal heart beats at a rate of 68 to 80 beats per minute in the adult, from 80 to 100 in the child, and from 110 to 130 in the infant. In the adult an increase to over 100 beats per minute is classified as "tachycardia," whereas a rate lower than 50 beats per minute is termed "bradycardia." As a general rule, tachycardia is a more common physiological response than bradycardia and is thus of less concern. Tachycardia may occur as a result of pain, emotion, exercise, or fever. The dentist should seek consultative advice before accepting as a patient anyone who has a resting pulse rate of more than 100 or less than 50.

The dentist should take and record the pulse as part of his pretreatment evaluation of each patient, noting its rate, rhythm, and volume. He should determine whether a tachycardia or bradycardia exists, whether the rhythm is regular or irregular, and whether the volume is bounding or soft. He should not attempt to diagnose an arrhythmia but must be aware of both its presence and its effect on the patient.

It is well to keep in mind the fact that a regular pulse is a luxury, not a necessity, and that many patients who are 40, 50, or older live normal, active lives despite existing arrhythmias. At this point, as in the case of the presence of a murmur, it is advisable to question the patient regarding his daily activities and work load. The patient with an arrhythmia who carries on an unimpeded daily schedule without duress should withstand dental treatment as well. Although practically every patient who is able to go about his daily activities without stress or strain, shortness of breath, or undue fatigue may be considered a satisfactory candidate for dental procedures, a patient who is subject to dyspnea or one who, because of inability to exert himself, leads a sedentary or inactive life will require special attention if dental procedures are to be tolerated satisfactorily. Stress, fear, and apprehension concerning the appointment should be controlled through the use of conscious-sedation.

RESPIRATORY STATUS

In general, alterations in the respiratory system do not produce such alarming results as may be found in the cardiovascular system. Nevertheless, some diseases of the respiratory system should be of interest to the dentist contemplating the use of conscious-sedation. Among these are (1) bronchitis, (2) bronchiectasis, (3) emphysema, and (4) asthma.

Bronchitis and bronchiectasis. The problems that patients with chronic bronchitis and bronchiectasis pose for the dentist are more annoying than hazardous. The common symptoms of these diseases include productive cough, dyspnea, and chest pain. Fetid breath may be present and may itself be a problem. The dentist should expect these patients to cough frequently and should plan his work accordingly. Having the patient cough well to clear the tracheobronchial tree immediately before work is begun, as well as scheduling the procedure for the afternoon rather than the morning, may help.

Emphysema. Pulmonary emphysema is a condition characterized by abnormal dilation of the terminal alveoli and other respiratory structures. Chronic emphysema is one of the most common forms of pulmonary disease. The state of the disease may range from a very mild form to a very severe, debilitating condition. The most common signs and symptoms of emphysema are dyspnea on exertion, cough, and in some cases cyanosis. As the disease progresses, the patient may exhibit a typical barrel-shaped chest and audible wheezes or deep breathing. When seeing an emphysematous patient in the office, the dentist should ascertain the extent of the disease. This is not difficult, since it is simply a matter of determining the degree of dyspnea, the frequency and severity of coughing spells, the occurrence of cyanosis, and—above all—the restricting effects of the disease on the patient's daily activities. Like the patient with bronchitis or bronchiectasis, the patient having emphysema should be asked to clear his tracheobronchial tree as well as possible just before dental work is started—by deep breathing and coughing. As a rule, early morning is not a good time for appointments; they should be scheduled for a time later in the day so that the patient will have had a chance to loosen and clear the lung fields.

The patient having a poor exercise tolerance will fare better during dental appointments if his fears and anxieties are relieved through the judicious use of conscious-sedation. Care must be exercised with the administration of any agents that may interfere with the cough reflex or depress an already compromised ventilation.

Asthma. Asthma, or bronchial asthma, is a pulmonary insufficiency brought on by spasmodic contraction of the bronchioles, which interferes with the passage of air into and out of the lungs. Exhalation is particularly difficult and prolonged, as compared to normal.

Some 50% or more of the cases of bronchial asthma are referred to as "extrinsic asthma"; those cases for which no allergen can be identified are usually the result of infections of the respiratory tract and are referred to as "intrinsic asthma."

In its most typical form asthma is a common disease and may be found in all age groups. Symptoms are usually sporadic, with ventilation being normal between attacks. Asthma may range from mild infrequent attacks to severe frequent ones. As with other entities, the dentist must determine not only the condition but also its frequency, its severity, and medications that may be in use for its treatment. When treating asthmatic patients, the dentist should avoid situations and conditions that tend to aggravate the disease. Among these are unexpected painful stimuli, irritating odors, exertion, and emotional episodes. For this reason asthmatic patients are particularly good candidates for conscious-sedation. With such aggravations eliminated, the patients will readily tolerate a contemplated dental procedure.

NERVOUS SYSTEM

Some diseases of the nervous system should be of interest to the dentist, since a knowledge of their presence would be of help in treatment and in selection of conscious-sedative procedures. Specifically, he should know if the patient is subject to (1) persistent headache or (2) convulsive disorders such as either grand mal epilepsy or petit mal epilepsy.

Persistent headache. During the pretreatment evaluation the dentist should be interested in the presence of persistent headaches; although they may be the result of tension, dissatisfactions, resentments, and so forth, they may also result from brain lesions or from hypertension. Pain is rarely referred from outside the head to the head area. One exception is that pain in the jaw region may be associated with coronary artery or anginal conditions.

An inquiry should be made of any patient with persistent headache to determine whether or not he is under the care of a physician and taking medication. If not, he should be referred to a physician for consultation after it has been determined that no oral cause exists. Unless it is specifically contraindicated, such a patient should be considered a prime candidate for conscious-sedation with regional analgesia during dental treatment.

Convulsive disorders. Convulsive disorders should always be of concern to the dentist, since they may alter the selection of drugs and pain control methods used. Grand mal and petit mal disorders are phenomena that may be produced by a variety of causes, with attacks occurring at indefinite times. A good history will inform the dentist of the type of seizure and the frequency of occurrence. Precipitating factors such as emotional stress, as well as the presence of auras that may precede the attack, may also be determined. It is also important to be aware of any medication that the patient is taking, and care should be taken to arrange for appointments at times when it is at its maximum effectiveness. It is important also to be certain that prescribed medication is being taken as directed.

In view of the fact that emotional episodes may trigger attacks, it is advisable to employ conscious-sedation with such an individual, to prevent a seizure from occurring. Barbiturates as well as certain psychosedatives are particularly useful in this regard.

METABOLIC DEFICIENCIES

The metabolic deficiencies of most interest to the dentist are (1) diabetes mellitus and (2) obesity.

Diabetes mellitus. The majority of patients having diabetes mellitus are aware of their condition and thus will give the information on the history. After learning that the patient is diabetic the dentist should ascertain the severity of his disorder. This is best accomplished by learning whether the patient controls his condition through diet alone, by oral hypoglycemic agents, or with insulin. A patient who controls his diabetes by diet, with or without oral hypoglycemic agents, should present no problems to the dentist. The patient who does require insulin should undergo dental treatment only between the hours of nine o'clock in the morning and twelve o'clock noon. It is during this period that he is best prepared to tolerate stressful situations. The patient should be instructed to take his insulin according to his usual regimen. Dental appointments should not be allowed to conflict with his meal schedule lest hypoglycemia, a greater concern than hyperglycemia, ensue. The diabetic patient tolerates medications well and may undergo conscious-sedation whenever the situation warrants it.

Obesity. Obesity is an accumulation of excess fat stored in the body. In extreme cases it deserves the attention that a serious disease demands. This condition may cause not only dyspnea and fatigue but also airway and cardiovascular problems. Thus cardiac and pulmonary problems often accompany extreme obesity. Many obese patients are emotional individuals, and their overeating is a form of psychological compensation. This is especially true of those patients who have experienced a recent and rapid weight gain. If one pursues the history of these patients, he frequently finds a psychologically traumatic event in their recent past. As a general rule, obese patients are much in need of conscious-sedation during dental appointments. However, they are usually difficult to manage from a technical aspect. Venipuncture may be difficult, if not impossible. Medication must be administered in amounts sufficient to meet the objectives, yet care must be taken to ensure that respiratory embarrassment will not occur.

ENDOCRINE IMBALANCES

The endocrine imbalances of most interest to the dentist include (1) hypothyroidism, (2) hyperthyroidism, and (3) adrenal insufficiency.

Hypothyroidism. A patient having hypothyroidism presents a typical appearance that usually make him easily recognizable. The skin is thick and dry. Perspiration rarely occurs. The hair is brittle and sparse, and he shows an increased sensitivity to cold temperatures. The patient usually has experienced recent weight gain and is edematous, and reactions are sluggish. Mental changes are present as well. Response to questioning is usually delayed and at times humorously inappropriate. All enzyme systems are underactive. This fact must be taken into account whenever conscious-sedation, using agents that require metabolic breakdown within the body, is employed.

Hyperthyroidism. In hyperthyroidism the patient appears anxious and restless and may be trembling. The skin is fine and the patient perspires excessively. In contrast to one with hypothyroidism, this patient tolerates a cold environment well and a warm one poorly. The heart rate is usually rapid and the individual complains of palpitations. Weight loss is present in spite of an increased appetite. Because of his anxious, restless behavior the hyperthyroid patient is a good candidate for conscious-sedation. Greater drug doses than would ordinarily be expected are frequently required to calm such a patient.

Adrenal insufficiency. In addition to being present in Addison's disease, a condition of adrenal insufficiency may be derived by either of the two mechanisms now discussed.

In the first, the patient has been exposed to a prolonged stressful situation such as a chronic and painful dental problem. The stress that the patient endures provokes the release of adrenal corticotropic hormone (ACTH) from the pituitary gland, which in turn stimulates the adrenal gland to release steroid hormones into the bloodstream. These hormones better enable the body's physiology to cope with the stressful situation. During periods of prolonged stress, however, the adrenal gland is overtaxed and cannot keep pace with the demands placed on it. As a result *adrenal exhaustion* occurs, and the patient's ability to tolerate stress decreases because there are insufficient circulating steroid hormones.

The second cause for adrenal insufficiency occurs as a result of the discontinuance of exogenously administered steroid hormones. Steroid hormone therapy decreases the output of ACTH from the pituitary gland. As a result endogenous steroid hormone production and release declines and the adrenal cortex *atrophies*. The atrophied gland is now unable to secrete hormones at a level sufficient to allow the patient to tolerate stressful situations well. This condition may prevail for as long as a month after the medication has been discontinued.

Regardless of the etiology of adrenal insufficiency, the patient has a diminished ability to tolerate stressful situations. Steroid hormones play an important role in the maintenance of normal blood pressure—particularly the ability to return a hypotensive state to a normotensive one.

Any patients suspected of having adrenal insufficiency should be medicated preoperatively with steroid hormones, to avoid problems of blood pressure maintenance. In addition, conscious-sedation should be employed to remove psychological stress that might precipitate a hypotensive episode. Narcotic analgetics are particularly useful for elevating the pain threshold and thus aiding in elimination of stress.

ALLERGIC MANIFESTATIONS

All patients must be questioned as to the presence of any allergies. While doing this, the dentist should bear in mind that there are "allergic-type" individuals. This means that the patient having multiple allergies—be these reactions to foods, pollens, drugs, or other materials—is more likely to be allergic or to become allergic to medication the practitioner may administer than is the "nonallergic" individual.

Characteristically, allergy is manifested primarily through the skin, mucous membranes, or blood vessels. It may be mild or severe and immediate or delayed (appearing up to 2 weeks or more after exposure to the allergen). Fortunately 95% of the allergic reactions seen in a dental office involve the skin and blood vessels, their form being a rash, hives, and itchiness.

The management of allergic manifestations is discussed in Chapter 11. Suffice it here to say that many patients are erroneously told that they are allergic to one drug or another by some practitioner who is at a loss to explain a particular episode. I have seen many patients who mistakenly reported having an allergy to Novocain because they "faint" when it is administered to them. Other patients of highly emotional makeup may develop a rash or hives when placed in surroundings that are unpleasant to them. Thus the appearance of such signs and symptoms while the patient is in a dental office may be misinterpreted as an allergic reaction. Good histories will usually enable the dentist to determine which of his patients are truly allergic individuals.

Conscious-sedation is not contraindicated in the allergic patient. However, drugs to which the patient may be allergic as well as any that are chemically related to possible allergens must be avoided.

MEDICATIONS THE PATIENT MAY BE TAKING

Because of advances in pharmacology, medicine, and related sciences many a patient owes his very life to the continued support he receives through pharmacotherapy. It is beyond the scope of this text to discuss the ramifications of such therapy for the myriad of drugs available. However, the importance of this aspect of the history must be stressed. The dentist must determine each patient's medication and its dosage—by consultation with the prescribing physician if necessary. He must then familiarize himself with all aspects of its pharmacology. Knowledge of medications will aid the history taken in discovering not only the condition for which the patient is being treated but also its severity.

Frequently, the patient may be taking drugs that will directly influence the conscious-sedative technique and choice of agents. Care must be taken to ensure that due consideration has been given to questions regarding possible synergistic or antagonistic effects.

HEMATOLOGICAL PATHOLOGIES

Although a tendency toward prolonged bleeding and delayed clotting is usually a surgical problem, it can be of concern also during the use of regional analgesia and venipuncture. The patient should be questioned during the history about any prolonged bleeding tendencies. It is also important to learn whether he has been receiving any anticoagulant therapy. In a patient taking any medication or having any condition that is likely to interfere with the clotting mechanism, deep regional injections in the area of a major vessel should be performed with caution, if at all.

Conscious-sedation might best be secured under these circumstances via the inhalation or oral routes. Intramuscular and intravenous injections may be used with caution. Care should be exercised to ensure as clean and atraumatic a venipuncture as possible.

IATROGENIC CONDITIONS

"Iatrogenic conditions" may be defined as physiological alterations resulting from a physician's treatment. This does not imply that the treatment is ill advised but indicates that certain medications and treatments may produce undesirable side effects. It is therefore essential that the dentist be so informed if the patient is under a physician's care and be told what medication, if any, the patient is taking. This knowledge will be of inestimable value for the following reasons:

1. It reduces the possibility of the dentist's giving any medication that may be incompatible with drugs prescribed by the physician.
2. It enables the dentist to avoid giving medications that may have either a potentiating or an additive effect with drugs prescribed by the physician.
3. It allows the dentist to avoid arranging appointments at a time of day not advantageous to the patient.
4. It enables the dentist to more knowingly consult with the physician for their mutual advantage and that of the patient.

PSYCHOLOGICAL AND EMOTIONAL INSTABILITY

All patients should be discreetly questioned about any previous unpleasant dental, medical, or anesthetic experiences. The effects in such experiences may have been caused by psychological or emotional instability rather than to any physical condition. A patient who is psychologically or emotionally unstable, is fearful or apprehensive, or has had an unpleasant experience will not tolerate the contemplated dental procedure well. However, if this patient's mood can be altered and his fear and apprehension eliminated through the use of conscious-sedation, he will become an excellent candidate for treatment under regional analgesia.

Certain aspects of the pretreatment evaluation are particularly useful in selecting these patients who, although physically healthy, are psychologically or emotionally distraught and may therefore be considered prime candidates for conscious-sedation. Some of the questions that, asked to each one, are particularly useful in selecting these patients will now be listed, with brief comments.

1. *What is your general state of health?* The patient who states that his general health is only fair or poor and complains of vague or nonspecific symptoms when the remainder of the pretreatment evaluation indicates that he is in good health is a good candidate for conscious-sedation. Such persons are overly concerned with their state of health, to the point that their psychological involvement dominates their lives. They are likely to be chronically complaining of minor disturbances while undergoing dental treatment. For their comfort and for the sake of efficiency on the part of the dentist, conscious-sedation is advisable.

2. *Are you now or have you recently been under the care of a physician? Are you now taking or have you taken any drugs recently?* These two questions may be discussed together, since they are relative to each other.

As mentioned earlier, those patients under the care of a physician and taking medications prescribed by him are frequently candidates for conscious-sedation, because of poor physical condition and inability to tolerate stressful situations. Many patients, however, are being treated for systemic disorders that are stress-induced or have psychosomatic origins. Ailments falling into this category include headache, asthma, gastric ulcers, irritable colon, and ulcerative colitis, to name a few.

Usually, these patients will be taking medications to control the symptoms exhibited, as well as a psychosedative or barbiturate. Since these patients are emotional, they are excellent candidates for conscious-sedation.

3. *Have you ever had a serious illness or operation?* In addition to determining the nature of the illness, so as to ascertain whether dental treatment must be altered, the dentist should question his patient regarding any anesthetic that has been administered. Those patients who have had unpleasant anesthetic experiences are prone to be fearful of conscious-sedation unless it is thoroughly explained to them. Recollection of a previous anesthetic may call up thoughts of nausea, vomiting, postoperative headache, and the like. Patients should be assured that conscious-sedation and general anesthesia are worlds apart and that unpleasant side effects are not likely to occur. In my experience I have seen only one or two properly prepared patients, out of thousands, become nauseated and none who has vomited following conscious-sedation.

A few patients are concerned that they will "talk" or "give away secrets" when conscious-sedation is employed. This may be related to events surrounding a previous general anesthetic or may be due to a movie or television program they have seen. They should be assured that this does not happen during conscious-sedation, since they will be awake at all times. I have never known this to occur in a patient during conscious-sedation—or while emerging from general anesthesia, for that matter.

4. *Have you ever had any shortness of breath?* Those apparently healthy patients who complain of shortness of breath are emotional individuals. They usually sigh frequently, a sign that the observant dentist will readily detect. They may relate that they frequently have difficulty "catching their breath" or may state that they "can't breathe," even while taking frequent deep breaths during the interview.

These individuals have difficulty taking a deep enough breath to satisfy a psychological need. Often they will take consecutive deep breaths until the need is finally satisfied. Their respiratory pattern will be normal for a period of time, only to return to the deep sighing pattern once again. Patients fitting this description stand to benefit greatly from use of conscious-sedation, as does the practitioner, since the bothersome respiratory pattern occurs most frequently in psychologically or emotionally disturbing situations. The dental appointment may well be such a situation.

5. *Have you ever been aware of a rapid heartbeat or palpitations?* The word *palpitation* merely means that the person is aware of his heartbeat. It does not connote any irregularity in rhythm or strength of the beat. Many laymen have this word in their vocabulary and will frequently relate that they "have palpitations." They may tell of a "sinking feeling" in the chest or state that the heart feels as if it "flops over" in the chest. Such persons may state that at night when they retire their heart is pounding so much that the entire bed seems to shake. In the absence of organic heart disease and other symptoms relating to the cardiovascular system, these patients may be considered to be emotional individuals. As such, they deserve the benefits of conscious-sedation during dental treatment.

6. *Are you troubled with frequent headaches?* Patients who are troubled with frequent headaches should be referred to a physician for evaluation if a dental origin for the headache cannot be found. In all probability, however, patients who are experiencing frequent headaches have already consulted a physician. In the absence of organic disease these patients may be considered to be emotional individuals. Careful questioning may demonstrate the occurrence of a headache in association with trying or stressful situations. Patients relating such histories should undergo conscious-sedation during dental treatment—to eliminate psychological stress and allow treatment to be rendered while they are comfortable and relaxed.

7. *Are you unduly apprehensive, fearful, or nervous?* Patients replying in the affirmative to this question are literally asking for some sort of assistance to help them through the dental visit. Those patients answering in the negative but obviously appearing to be nervous and upset are doing likewise. The apprehensive, nervous patient is not very good at hiding his anxiety. He may sigh or wet his lips frequently, tap his fingers or feet, and move restlessly and look about anxiously, rather than look at the history taker. This example again points out the need for observation and careful listening by the dentist while taking the history. In spite of his behavior, the patient may state that he is not apprehensive. Conscious-sedation should be employed in patients of this type if the chair time is to be productive for both patient and practitioner.

8. *Have you ever consulted a psychiatrist?* Those patients who now are or previously have been under the care of a psychiatrist are obviously psychologically disturbed. Careful attention must be paid to make sure that the dental visit does not add additional psychological stress for a patient who is little able to tolerate it. If psychiatric help was sought because of drug or alcohol dependence, consultation with the patient's psychiatrist may be in order lest the dentist choose medications for conscious-sedation that may interfere with the progress of treatment. Generally speaking, a patient who is under psychiatric care will fare better during dental treatment if conscious-sedation is employed.

9. *Have you had any recent weight gain?* As mentioned earlier, the obese patient usually is of an emotional makeup. The same may be said about the patient who, while not obese, has experienced a rapid and recent weight gain. By questioning closely, the dentist will usually be able to uncover a psychologically traumatic event in the recent past. Such events as the loss of a loved one, financial problems, and so forth are not uncommon in the patient experiencing recent weight gain. As with other emotional patients, conscious-sedation should be employed during dental treatment.

10. *Do your hands sweat excessively?* One sure sign that the patient is fearful and concerned over impending dental treatment is the presence of perspiration on the palms of the hands. Often, the patient will deny the presence of such a finding. But, on shaking hands or offering assistance into the office, the dentist will frequently notice the presence of moist palms. Although this may be associated with pathological states, in the absence of other positive findings moist hands generally indicate that the patient is a bit fearful and thus a good candidate for conscious-sedation.

11. *Are you easily fatigued?* This question, like many others, may indicate the presence of a systemic disorder. However, in the absence of other significant findings it may reveal that the practitioner is dealing with an emotional patient, particularly if fatigue is sudden in onset and unexplained in cause. The individual should thus be considered as emotional in type and receive the benefits of conscious-sedation throughout the course of dental treatment.

12. *Do you smoke? Do you drink?* Not all patients who use tobacco and/or alcohol are emotional individuals. However, a great many of the persons who do have one of these habits will be using it as a psychological or emotional crutch. The patient who smokes one cigarette after another while nervously moving about is not smoking for the enjoyment. The individual who imbibes alcohol just prior to visiting the dental office is not drinking to be "sociable."

Under these circumstances a habit is being used to aid the individual through a psychologically trying yet physically necessary episode. These persons also should be considered as fearful, emotional patients and good candidates for dentistry under regional analgesia plus conscious-sedation. However, it is not advisable to undertake dental treatment in the individual who has consumed alcohol prior to visiting the office. The use of conscious-sedation in this patient is particularly unwarranted, since almost all agents employed will have their effects enhanced by the presence of alcohol.

Needless to say, the possible mechanisms for the recognition of the patient with a psychological or emotional problem have not been exhausted. Many patients will present with more than one sign or symptom relative to their emotional status. The goal of the examiner must be to evaluate and integrate all pertinent findings so that the patient's emotional status and his need for conscious-sedation may be placed in its proper perspective.

SUMMARY

Once again the importance of the pretreatment evaluation prior to dental procedures must be emphasized. Not only does it permit the dentist to determine the patient's physical and psychological ability to tolerate the stress of the dental visit, but it also enables him to prepare for the appointment by proper scheduling and allotment of chair time. It enables him to determine the need for conscious-sedation and allows him to select the technique, drugs, and route of administration best suited to each patient. The pretreatment evaluation should serve as a guide that can be followed to determine how a particular patient must be managed. As a general rule, the greater the patient's deviations from normal and the poorer his exercise tolerance, the greater is the indication for conscious-sedation.

Chapter 4

ANXIETY IN THE DENTAL OFFICE

Robert E. Pearson

Many people express astonishment on first discovering that over half of the population of the United States regularly, determinedly, and actively avoid regular, professional dental care. Eyebrows go even higher when it is stated that most of those individuals stay away from the dental office because they are afraid that they are going to be hurt. After all, the modern dentist has many techniques available to make his patients comfortable. There is really no good reason for a person to avoid caring for something as vital to his health as his teeth and mouth.

Those are good and meaningful comments, but they come most often from someone who is more used to having a drill in his hand than in his mouth.

Normal human beings do not like to experience pain. They do not even like to *think* about pain. But they do so. They think about pain they have had in the past and are concerned about pain they may have in the future. It is part of normal human development to learn early and thoroughly what kind of situation is likely to result in physical and emotional discomfort and then avoid such situations as much as possible in the future.

Pain or a threat of pain to the mouth area is particularly frightening to most of us, because the mouth is an extremely important part of the body. All theories of human personality development have to acknowledge in one way or another the importance of the mouth. In the infant this is the first area brought under conscious control. Nourishment is taken in or rejected. Emotions are expressed, such as smiling, crying, and scowling. Vocal language is well developed before the child can control his bladder or bowels. The world is actually felt and tasted before it is seen.

Another lesson we all learn as very young children is that something that hurts is not functioning properly or maybe will not function at all. It really is easy to understand why the threat of pain to this area of unequaled importance results in anxiety.

The education of those who never go to a dentist, for whatever reasons, is beyond the scope of this discussion. Undoubtedly the best hope of making a significant impact on this group lies in the area of education of the children. The main thrust of this chapter will be to discuss the worries and fears of those people who do manage to visit a dentist but who are also unhappy about it.

CAUSES OF ANXIETY

From this point forward, the use of the word "anxiety" will be confined to that which occurs in the dental office. This particular anxiety, probably present to some degree in almost everyone who sits in "that chair," has in its more severe form been called a phobia, or even a "dentophobia." But a phobia is defined as an *unreasonable* fear, usually displaced from something else, which is really feared unconsciously. I submit that the anxiety is not entirely unreasonable, and that the patient knows perfectly well what he is anxious about. Anxiety is a learned response, learned either from past personal experience or from the experience of others. It is felt in anticipation of the occurrence of something unpleasant. Anxiety is a common occurrence in dental patients because they feel something unpleasant *might* happen.

Personal experience is usually the most effective teacher. One strongly unpleasant experience, especially in childhood, can establish an automatic fright response to the same *or similar* experiences in the future. These responses can last a lifetime. Among my own memories is one of feeling absolutely certain that I was about to die—the result of what was probably a poorly administered nitrous oxide anesthetic. The gas certainly could not have been administered for more than 3 minutes; but even now, almost 45 years later, it seems unlikely that I could be persuaded to receive nitrous oxide again.

Very often the sensitizing event or events will be distorted or completely forgotten, but the result will be the same. Having the patient recall events that may be responsible for his anxiety can sometimes be helpful but is usually quite time-consuming, difficult, and uncertain; also (happily) this is *almost never necessary*. Other effective methods that require less time are available.

Another reason for dental anxiety is that it is *expected* of us! How many people would admit that they do not mind going to the dentist? Our culture, through parents, peers, and the inundation of television and other one-way communicators, teaches us that one should have at least some dislike for psychiatrists, dentists, spinach, mothers-in-law, and the Internal Revenue Service.

One method people use to control their own anxiety is to laugh at the things they fear—witness the countless jokes and cartoons about dentists, psychiatrists, and the I.R.S. How many times are these subjects portrayed on television as characters to be laughed at? The writers of one television comedy series knew their audience well; their main character was a psychotherapist and the "second banana" a dentist.

People are also anxious when they are uncertain as to just what is going to happen to them. There are certain procedures in dentistry that *never* have been painful, yet people often react to having radiographs taken, having their teeth *looked* at, etc., as if something terrible is happening. Much anxiety can be markedly lessened by explaining precisely, in words that a nondentist can easily understand, what is happening now, how much, if any, discomfort will be felt, and how long it will last. If the practitioner will do that with all his patients, he will quickly come to be thought of as a concerned human being, and one could hardly wish for better than that!

The role of the dentist in causing anxiety

Anxiety is also similar in many respects to a contagious disease; people catch it from other people and then pass it on to still others who have not been "vaccinated." The incubation period is very short, and if untreated the disease may last a lifetime.

Quite obviously patients catch this disease from other patients in spite of all attempts by the dental profession to keep the infection from spreading. Right?

Not quite.

Anxiety is also spread by dental practitioners who, if not usually the primary source of infection, often make mild cases worse. It would seem to be obvious that at least one of the participants in a therapeutic relationship should be at ease; yet this is not always the case. Many physicians and dentists have never learned to be comfortable in relating to patients and, in turn, transmit a discomfort to them. I believe that we doctors have a perfectly adequate reason for being uncomfortable with patients: we were taught it in medical and dental school. Please note that I used the word "reason," not "excuse." Only recently have more than a few schools begun to deal with teaching students to be comfortable in their roles as healers.

I remember well how I was taught to be uncomfortable with patients. After literally hundreds of hours spent in hearing lectures on physical diagnosis and history taking, and in practicing on other students, I was told by an instructor to go to Room ABC and do a history and physical on the patient I would find there. Five minutes later the patient and I were both wondering what in the world was going on. When I told the instructor of my discomfort, I was told not to worry about it, since learning to be comfortable with a patient was just a matter of being with one enough times. I learned many things in medical school that turned out later to be not true, but that was the biggest lie of them all!

Some students remain so chronically uncomfortable when they are with patients that they decide to go into a specialty that requires little or no direct patient contact. A few even drop out of school. Still others become so alternately enraged and challenged that they go into psychiatry, only to find that even there (some would say *especially* there) the professional helpers are often not at ease with those seeking the help.

Please pause here for a moment and, using a word or a short phrase, answer this question to yourself: *What are you?*

When I have asked that question before large groups, people have seemed strangely upset by it. Some say that the question is too silly to bother with—the answer is so obvious that they need not respond—or they laugh, look wise, and wait for someone else to answer. A professional person will often answer the question by saying that he is a physician, a dentist, a teacher, a psychiatrist, a surgeon, or the like.

I submit that the best possible answer to the question is that you are *a human being living among other human beings.* I believe that the reason we think as so many of us do is that during our training we were somehow brainwashed into believing that the *roles* we play as human beings are what we *really are.*

The other answers given (physician, dentist, etc.) are only concrete descriptions of temporary roles we play as human beings. Sometimes, like effective actors, we get so absorbed in playing an allotted role that we forget what and who we really are. When we become deluded that we are the characters shown in the roles we are playing, we tend to do things *to* patients, including occasionally using patients to fulfill our own needs instead of theirs. Sometimes we have a better opinion of ourselves and imagine ourselves doing things *for* patients. As human beings we should think of ourselves as doing things *with* patients.

The point of this discussion is that if we can relearn and think of ourselves as human beings, each of us playing a temporary role as a practitioner of a healing art, it would be much easier to relate to that other human being who is temporarily playing the role of patient. Doctors, like everyone else, become anxious when they feel that they are being threatened. "People" are really much less threatening than "patients."

Our patients are not really out to give us a bad time and make things difficult for us, although that idea seems to be a chronic delusion for many of us. They are often merely responding to the tensions they sense in the doctor. If we can learn to play our roles comfortably, recognizing that they *are* roles, almost all of our patients will learn to play their roles comfortably also.

RECOGNITION OF ANXIETY

So far this discussion has been mainly concerned with some of the causes of anxiety. Some introductory comments on the subject of management will be made shortly, and in Chapter 5 discussion includes several methods of managing the anxious dental patient. However, the anxious patient must be recognized before he can be effectively treated, so now I will discuss how one might go about determining which patients are anxious enough to warrant the use of special techniques. Some patients do say to their dentist, "I'm afraid of what you're going to do to me, and I want help in this area," but they are rare. Most anxious patients try to "grin and bear it" one way or another, so the dentist will have to be looking for signs that indicate undue tension.

First of all, the receptionist or hygienist can be invaluable in spotting the anxious patient. Patients will often say things to the dental auxiliary or in their presence that they would not dream of saying to the dentist. The practitioner's aides know much better than he does how his various patients behave in the reception room. Asking these assistants to help identify the frightened patients will both improve the dentist's image with his aides and will also allow all to be more comfortable in their roles.

Anxious people frequently break appointments and are particularly prone to do this at the last minute. Something else is always erupting in their lives to justify not going to the dentist yet. One advantage of this ploy is that they can continue to tell themselves and the world how hard they have been trying to get that dental work done. With a few variations on the theme, such as forgetting a few appointments or asking for an appointment when the dentist is on vacation, they manage to delay the confrontation for many years, the anxiety mounting with the passage of each broken appointment. In other cases the patient may hesitate seating himself in the dental chair and once in it will keep moving about seeking a comfortable position, one he never does seem able to find.

Much can be learned from a patient's voice—not only through what his words say but also by the tone he uses. The dentist should listen carefully; he will learn a great deal, even if he does not think he will. Most people have little confidence in their ability to judge another person's mood by the sound of that person's voice, but everyone can do it. This really should not surprise us. After all, as an infant each of us responded to the tone of his mother's voice long before he realized that the individual sounds she was making had meanings of their own. Bravado is *always* a cover-up for fears of some kind. Tremulousness has an obvious meaning; some people refuse to speak if they suspect that their voice will be shaky.

The dentist should observe how the patient positions himself in the dental chair. Are more than occiput, elbows, and heels touching something? Are the eyes, mouth, and fists all clenched? Perhaps *all* orifices are being held tightly closed? One should at least suspect that the patient is not enjoying himself.

Teeth that obviously have not had professional care for a long time are a reliable indicator of underlying anxiety about dentistry.

Anxiety often is seen in the questions a patient asks. Not only: "Is it going to hurt much?" but also "What is that for? I haven't seen that before. What do you do with that?" etc. Such questions often can be translated into: "Please tell me that I'm not going to make a fool of myself." Questions are also used to repeatedly delay or interrupt the dentistry itself. Here they serve the same function as coughing, unnecessary gagging, having to rinse the mouth, and all the other ploys every dentist knows so well.

It is extremely important to assess the anxiety level of each patient. With a minimum of practice the dentist will be seeing things he has never noticed before.

As mentioned in Chapter 3, the pretreatment history and physical evaluation constitute an invaluable tool to aid in the recognition of the anxious and apprehensive dental patient. Numerous physical manifestations—frequent sighing, tachycardia, blood pressure changes, etc.—are reliable indications of not only the presence of anxiety but its degree as well. Careful pretreatment evaluation coupled with close patient observation will be rewarded many times over for the minimum amount of time required.

MANAGEMENT OF ANXIETY

Simple recognition of anxiety is obviously not enough. Something must be done with and about that knowledge. As a matter of fact, it is impossible to not respond to the patient's message; even ignoring the message is one way of responding to it. If you do not at least acknowledge that you recognize that he is uncomfortable, he will be forced to assume that you have not heard his message (you are stupid), that you have heard it and don't care (you are unfeeling), or that you have heard it and he is correct in believing he has reason to be frightened.

With most anxious patients the appropriate thing is to say something such as "You seem a bit tense—do you feel tense?" or "How can I help you with it?"

It is always astonishing to see how patients grasp at remarks that show concern, and that that type of remark is all that many patients need to alleviate their fears.

Patients not amenable to this simple approach will, in all probability, be excellent candidates for the conscious-sedative techniques discussed in other sections of this text. Through the use of conscious-sedation, patients will not only be relieved of their anxieties during the current dental treatment; many will also come to realize that dentistry need not be the frightening experience it once was *"expected"* to be! Thus, through the use of this adjunct to pain and apprehension control, many patients will have their unfounded fears eliminated and will be able to undergo future dental procedures without the need for pharmacological assistance. That is to say, many may be weaned from any necessity for having all future dental procedures performed with the use of conscious-sedation. Others will benefit from the use of conscious-sedative procedures at each dental office visit.

A fringe benefit to be gained from the use of pain and apprehension control modalities discussed in this text is that they serve as a means to educate the individual who fails to seek dental care primarily out of fear—fear related either to past personal experience or to something learned from the experience of others. Just as many potential dental patients have learned to fear the dentist, proper patient management through the use of conscious-sedation may serve to educate or reeducate these same individuals to the modern concept of dental practice. Friends and relatives of those patients who have undergone dental treatment with the use of conscious-sedation will soon learn of its merits. Hearing of a dental procedure that was accomplished painlessly while the patient was in a conscious, comfortable, and relaxed state may serve to dispel anxiety in many of the potential dental patients who now fail to seek dental care, out of fear alone.

SUMMARY

It is imperative that the practicing dentist become acutely aware of the pain and apprehension control needs of patients if dental care is to be efficiently and effectively administered to all who request or require it. One must realize the other causes of anxiety as well as gain an appreciation for his own role in its propagation and in its control. He must become knowledgeable and proficient in the use the tools—pretreatment evaluation and careful patient observation—that are used to recognize those patients in need of some form of anxiety control assistance. Finally, the practitioner must become thoroughly familiar with all useful means in the management of the anxious dental patient.

Above all, the dentist must know his role in the doctor-patient relationship. In this respect, I feel that good training in the use of suggestion and hypnosis would prove invaluable. To be effective in the use of these modalities the practitioner *must* play a role (that of the operator), which forces him to respond to the needs of the patient and to relate on a person-to-person basis.

Some practitioners may learn the techniques of hypnosis and then never put a patient into a trance, but even they find that learning the attitudes and approach to the patient that characterize a good operator improves their relationship with patients.

They learn to play the role of a sensitive concerned human being, who knows how to play his role as therapist comfortably and who can teach another human being (the patient) to be as comfortable as possible in playing his role.

As many of us can testify, finding and handling difficult problems can be a challenge and can even be fun. What more could any human being, whose role is dentist, ask?

Chapter 5

THE ROLE OF SUGGESTION IN PAIN AND ANXIETY CONTROL

Kay F. Thompson

Dentistry is surrounded by endless opportunities for service, and part of the satisfaction of being a dentist should be the reward of meeting the needs of the patients. With the current emphasis on dental health, more people than ever should be willing to seek dental care. What happens after they "go to a dentist" determines to a large extent whether they will return.

Although dentistry changes and becomes more sophisticated, the patient's problems change very little. Fear—almost a phobia—concerning dental treatment is widespread. If dentists are to offer a total service, they must have some understanding of this problem. A practice that manages to control the flow of traffic, sterilization of instruments, patient schedules, and office routine must also include the use of suggestion to help patients respond positively to dental treatment. No matter how well a practice is regulated, a neurotic, apprehensive, and/or phobic patient can upset a schedule—and one's disposition. Unless all such patients are to be eliminated from one's practice, a basic understanding of the psychology of patient management must be within the province of every dentist.

Dentists have usually been taught to expect patients to be frightened and uncomfortable, but they have not been taught how to allay this fear and discomfort. The use of various medications plays an integral part in the management of these patients, but sometimes a knowledge of sedatives and anesthetics is not enough. As one patient put it when she came in for extraction of four impacted third molars, "I know you can take care of the physical pain; it is the psychological pain I am concerned about."

The dentist works in the field of iatrogenic health. The properly oriented dentist can create a healthy situation where an unhealthy one previously existed, although, according to Erickson,* the dentist must be psychodynámi-cally oriented if he is to treat patients with neurotically disposed ideas of dentistry. Occasionally the dentist will learn that he can make *some* patients more comfortable by the things he says and does than by the medication he uses.

THE LANGUAGE OF SUGGESTION—VERBAL AND NONVERBAL COMMUNICATION

An attempt will be made here to consider some of the remarks that are said or might be said, as well as some that are better left unsaid during work with dental patients. The examples given are simply examples. It is hoped that they may encourage the dentist to scrutinize his approach to his own individual patients and develop a more comfortable way of delivering certain information to them.

The dentist can and must tell patients what is involved in their treatment, but he can do so in language that will not increase apprehension. This will require that he have some understanding of the attitudes of his patients, which can only be gained by listening to them. Hayakawa has spoken of listening as follows:

> The purpose of a conference is, of course, the exchange of ideas . . . (it is) a situation created specifically for the purposes of communication. There are two aspects to communication. One is the manner of output. But the other aspect of communication, namely, the problem of intake—especially the problem of how to listen well—is relatively a neglected subject. A common difficulty . . . is what might be called the "terminological tangle" in which discussion is stalemated by conflicting definitions of key terms. Listening means trying to see the problem the way the speaker sees it—which means not sympathy, which is "feeling for" him, but empathy, which is "experiencing with" him. Listening requires entering actively and imaginatively into the other fellow's situation and trying to understand a frame of reference different from your own. This is not always an easy task.†

The patient's acceptance of dentistry is the most important aspect of dental practice, for without it there would be no one on whom to utilize the mechanical skills learned in dental school. A dental practice is composed of at least two people, the dentist and the patient, working toward a mutual goal—the patient's adjustment to living.

It is difficult for patients to judge the quality of dentistry; it is frequently on some personal impression that their decisions are based. It is, then, the interpersonal relationship that influences patients to accept or reject dental care. How does the dentist motivate his patients to accept routine ministrations matter-of-factly, without fear and apprehension?

---

*Erickson, M. H. (Pittsburgh, Pa.):Personal communication, 1968.
†From Hayakawa, S. I., editor: The use and misuse of language, Greenwich, Conn., 1962, Fawcett Publishers, Inc., p. 73. Used by permission of the author.

The practitioner of dentistry constantly uses suggestions, some good and some bad, that affect his patients' attitudes. These suggestions, if only properly utilized, could help the patient to relax and enjoy good dentistry. The effective use of language in suggestion has already been mentioned. Such management begins with the creation of the proper impression on the patient in his first overt contact with the dental office. In all probability he had formed a tentative opinion prior to the time he called the office—this dentist may have been recommended by a respected friend and is said to be a "good" dentist, an "understanding" dentist, or a "painless" dentist. Hopefully, not too many patients choose a dentist today by picking a name at random from the yellow pages of the telephone book.

During his professional study, the dentist has been told that receptionists should be instructed to answer the telephone "with a smile," to help reassure the frightened patient and to start building a favorable image of the dentist. The voice of a pleasant, kind, and considerate receptionist will assist the dentist in gaining the trust and confidence of his patients.

Motivation and reassurance are further reinforced by nonverbal communication in the reception room and office. The room in which a patient must wait should be cheerful, warm, and up-to-date in decor as well as reading material. A neat, well-organized, and scrupulously clean office is also an integral part of nonverbal communication.

On his arrival at the office the patient should not be kept waiting without having his presence acknowledged. This would tend to demonstrate disregard for him as an individual. If, due to unforeseen circumstances, the patient must wait longer than anticipated, a brief statement to the effect that "the doctor will see you shortly" is in order. Statements such as "the doctor is having a difficult time with this extraction, but he will be with you shortly" are to be avoided. Although no actual contact with the person of the doctor has been made, definite impressions of the practitioner, be they favorable or unfavorable, are made by such statements.

Nonverbal communication is a continuous factor in the doctor-patient contact. The doctor should greet the patient warmly, perhaps with a handshake, thereby expressing his friendship, kindness, and sincerity. This also gives him the opportunity to observe the patient for clues concerning his emotional state. Is the hand hot, cold, clammy, hesitant, secure? Behavior during the remainder of the appointment continues to impart information.

Whether there is anything really difficult for a patient about sitting down in the dental chair will depend on his previous experiences, as well as his future expectations!

Unspoken attitudes and attentions by the dentist, as he quietly adjusts the headrest or offers a "tissue," express care and reassurance better than any spoken word. For the dentist who argues that these actions are too time-consuming in a busy practice, it should be pointed out that once a patient learns that he can trust the dentist to keep him comfortable dental work can be accomplished much more quickly and efficiently. Spending with a patient the amount of time that one would normally wait for a local anesthetic to take effect can, on occasion, be more rewarding than the anesthetic itself.

By the nature of his profession the dentist is often forced to perform difficult and sometimes painful procedures. Patients should therefore be given as much support as possible to help them tolerate such work. Some will respond best to encouragement, others to explanation, still others to direction and guidance. No matter which is chosen, it must be remembered that patients are people. Correct semantics, good operating technique, a considerate approach, and simple explanations of the procedures are often all that is required by the patient. Most people are capable of integrating their fears quite well. Fear of the unknown causes anxiety. Once the unknown is known and understood, an ability to tolerate it can usually be developed. By accepting these as possibilities and thus communicating with patients the dentist can enhance mutual goals.

Semantics. Careful attention to semantics should be recognized as one of the most effective tools to be used as a part of verbal communication. Dentistry utilizes many words that are alarming. Words such as cut, cauterize, hurt, pain, needle, inject, suture, extract, drill, and scalpel are all negative words. Even the term "operatory" may be distressing to some patients. There is another group of words that we often use without pay attention to their implications. These include such terms as the following: after, if, not until, whether, when, before, as long as, etc. If we say to a patient, "Tell me *when* it hurts," we are implying that the procedure *will* hurt; his function is simply a matter of discriminating *when* the pain can be felt. This can be replaced by saying, "If you think any of this procedure might bother you, raise your hand and I will stop." This gives the patient permission to stop the dentist at any time he feels apprehensive and thus gives him control over the situation. The new patient may need to test the dentist once or twice, but *when* he learns that he can trust his dentist he can relax and be comfortable.

Most patients are concerned about anticipated pain for a number of reasons. They do not know what kind of pain to expect, nor do they know how long it will last. They are concerned about possibly losing self-control and becoming embarrassed. Many persons can tolerate discomfort if they know it will last for only a few seconds or some other specified period of time. Being sure to inform patients and thereby giving them a degree of control over the situation reduces these fears.

Consider the patient who is usually disturbed by the thought of needles and injections. Appropriate explanations and careful technique can help alleviate this apprehension. Most dental students learn that injections should be given slowly and gently, but too many practitioners consider injections something to perform as rapidly as possible, to avoid wasting time. Topical anesthetics *do* help, but only if they are given time to become effective. The use of disposable needles has almost eliminated the problem of dull needles as well as the possibility of infection, and using sharp needles can eliminate almost entirely the discomfort associated with needle insertion. Once the topical anesthetic is applied, a half minute or so should be allowed to pass for the solution to reach maximal effectiveness. After the topical solution anesthetizes that tissue area, needle insertion can be completed slowly and painlessly. As this is being done, the dentist reassures the patient by reminding him to breathe deeply and easily and to stay relaxed and so notice how much simpler this was than he had really expected it to be.

Distraction. With a patient who does not seem to be able to relax there is a one-time approach that can be utilized. A direction of unexpected type is intended to distract the patient. For example, just as the mandibular injection is begun, the patient may be told, in a firmly directive voice, something such as "Now, relax your belly button!" As the patient registers the words and their incongruity and tries to figure out what response is expected, the injection is made without the patient noticing. After the injection has been completed, it is possible to point out the effectiveness of the distraction technique and convince the patient that injections are nothing to fear. This works only once, but once is usually enough.

Working with children. With very young children or those individuals who have never experienced a local anesthetic injection, the procedure can be even simpler. Repetition is usually nonthreatening, as the patient knows what is going to happen. By applying a topical anesthetic with a cotton applicator the dentist can turn back and forth a few times for additional liquid. One of those times the dentist can turn back with the syringe. The child is accustomed to the routine, so that the point of the needle can be inserted into the tissue painlessly while the fingers can obstruct the patient's clear view of the entire injection procedure. The child must be made to understand that his teeth will "go to sleep" while the cavities are removed from his teeth. He must also be told that his mouth *will* wake up again, and that he must not chew his cheek or tongue while they are asleep or they will be sore when they wake up. Handing the child a mirror, to demonstrate that his face is not swollen and that he looks the same, will alleviate a normal fear response to a strange feeling.

Children who are introduced to dental procedures in this thoughtful manner do *not* mature into adults who are terrified of dentistry. Children need to determine what kind of individual the dentist is and whether he is trustworthy. Providing a mirror for the child to watch the procedures may be beneficial in this area also. The message conveyed is "If he's willing to let me watch what he is doing, it must not be going to be that bad." The side benefit of the mirror is that the child becomes interested in the activity in the mirror and does not pay attention to the procedures actually being performed in his mouth. This is a pretend game, and children are experts at pretending.

A primary requisite for working with children in dentistry or in any other field is flexibility. If the child can be allowed to actively participate when it is practical, then when it is necessary for him to be still and cooperate, he will take his turn at that. Children can be a delight in dental practices, but only if one gains their friendship and cooperation and merits their trust. With fairness children will accept the limitations of the office and the firmness occasionally exhibited by the dentist.

Examples and effects of communication. The prestige and authority of the dentist have much to do with the way the patient responds to treatment. Dentists should therefore pay particular attention to their verbal and nonverbal communication. The dentist might say, "I'll have to give you a shot for this; it is a very deep cavity and will be difficult and would be painful without one." Or he might say, "It appears that there will be a reasonable amount of preparation to get this cavity into the right shape for restoring the tooth. You will be more comfortable if you have an anesthetic, so that neither of us will have to wonder if it might bother you as I work." If the patient responds, "I don't want Novocain" the dentist *could* reply, "OK, but don't say I didn't warn you." Or he *might* say, "That's fine, we can go ahead without an anesthetic, but if you decide at any time that you would prefer having one, we can always use it." Without an anesthetic the conversation might go, "You know, there is a lot of old amalgam to remove here. Big fillings usually mean that the blood vessels and nerve in the tooth have had an opportunity to pull back into the tooth so that the tooth is less sensitive. By the time I remove this old amalgam filling, which of course has no feeling in it, there won't be much left to do. The tooth has more or less prepared itself." or he *might* say, "We are almost finished now, and you have done very well with all these feelings and pressures. The tooth is beginning to look healthy." The entire procedure may also be interspersed with "Humms" and frowns, with slow thorough examination of the internal structure and much head shaking. The alternate approach is to make positive comments about any progress, reassuring the patient that the procedure is moving along nicely.

If the cavity preparation is in reality an especially difficult one, the dentist must explain to this patient what to expect. He can warn the patient about the seriousness of the situation by saying, "Mrs. Jones, that was a very deep cavity, with so much decay in it that before I finally got it all cleaned out I could see the pulp chamber showing through the dentin. I'm not too sure this tooth is going to be all right, so I'm not going to put in a permanent filling, I'm going to try a temporary one. We can then wait a while to see whether the tooth will flare up. If it starts to bother you at all, don't wait, call me right away." How much better to say, "Mrs. Jones, we have the decay removed and your tooth is nice and clean. You know that metals conduct heat and cold. If I put a metal restoration in your tooth right now, it would have those kinds of temperature reactions. I am going to put in a sedative cement that is soothing to the nerve and will give the blood vessels and nerve tissue a chance to draw back away from the area of the restoration. Later I can remove only the top part of this cement and replace it with a permanent metal restoration. We will make your appointment for this right now. In the meantime, this should feel pretty normal in your mouth. If you have any questions about it, please call me."

With the first approach the patient will probably go home and think about what she has been told. Her tongue will start to explore the tooth and as the anesthetic wears off she will wonder if that is how it should feel. She will wonder whether it will hurt whenever she eats or drinks anything hot or cold. As she becomes more alarmed, her emotions take over and she wonders whether the tooth hurts—yet. What can she do? Call the dentist! In the second case the patient does not anticipate difficulty. It is the responsibility of the patient to report anything unusual; it is the responsibility of the dentist to determine what action to take.

The dentist who is willing to make the effort to explain to his patient what he is doing can help the patient in his understanding of dentistry. Each time the dentist reaches for a new instrument, picks up the "drill" again, or starts, stops, looks carefully, and then changes something, the patient wonders, "What now?" It is very reassuring for the patient to be kept informed. Mild explanatory comments can be made at intervals, and deliberately: "There, that's cleaned out nicely"; "We're about half done now"; "Just a minute more and this wall will be straightened"; "You are such an excellent patient it makes my work easier"; "All we do now is smooth the edges," etc. Minor sensations can also be acknowledged: "I know you feel that pressure; the gum tissue on the cheek side of the tooth is not supposed to be numb"; "The suction as we remove the impression will feel as though your teeth are coming too"; "You can feel that tooth moving back and forth as I compress the tissues around it to provide more room," etc.

When speaking about impressions one might make comments such as "This impression material has a nice flavor—sassafras, I think; it will be ready to remove in x minutes;" or "This is an excellent impression material and has almost no taste, but it's an interesting color. In only 5 minutes it will be ready to remove" (not "set up," like plaster); or "When I remove this, it will feel as though everything in your mouth will come, too, but I promise you it won't." These comments reassure the patient that what he is feeling is what all patients are expected to feel.

The patient also needs an opportunity to understand that something that hurt him or frightened him before need not do so again. Anxiety can be reduced by a combination appeal to both logic and emotion, particularly if there is confidence in the person doing the persuading. A patient may respond to the following rationale: "Look, you are still very frightened of the dentist, possibly from something that happened a long time ago. You realize that many things have happened since then and that many changes have occurred. When you go back to visit the house in which you grew up, the rooms do not seem as big and bright as they once did. The hill out back where you played 'King of the Mountain' is not a mountain anymore; it's just a hill. The sizes really haven't changed, but the way you look at them has been altered. The unpleasant dental experience you had a long time ago is one you are still looking at through the eyes of long ago, and that is not fair. Other things have changed; you have grown up and altered your opinions and reactions toward many things; it is time to change your attitudes toward dentistry, too. It is not right to let something that happened such a long time ago influence your entire future. Give yourself a chance. Times and techniques have improved and you might be pleasantly surprised to find that dentistry can be a comfortable, ordinary, normal experience." If the dentist continues to verbalize additional helpful instruction, the patient may begin to adopt a new attitude.

One of the most threatening procedures in dentistry can be oral surgery. The patient may recognize that the removal of a tooth is essential for his health, but this does not mean that he wants to have it done. He may feel sorry about the loss of a part of *him,* just as he would if he were losing a gallbladder or an appendix. His fear frequently leads him to request a general anesthetic, so that he can be "asleep" and not know anything about what happens. Reassurance about the procedure may persuade the patient to have the extraction with a local anesthetic, which often is more appropriate than general anesthesia. Explanation of tooth removal should include the fact that the tooth is encased in a socket edged by a cartilaginous substance that is somewhat like the end of the nose. Compressing this substance allows room for an instrument to be slipped in beside the tooth, to pop it out. With a more difficult extraction one might mention the fact that the bone is very solid around the tooth, and that some of it will be removed to make the procedure simpler. The tooth may be removed in one piece; or it may be best to section it, enabling pieces to be removed more easily separately. These explanations will account for the noises to be heard during the time before the tooth is removed. The patient might be made to understand that more time is involved in this kind of extraction, but that it is a simple thing, and that healing occurs much faster. The patient should be reassured both during and after the extraction that he was a fine cooperative patient. He might be told: "Since you stayed so comfortable and relaxed, bleeding and disruption of the tissues were minimal. This permits the circulation to be very active in that area, and new cells will quickly replace the ones that were disturbed during the extraction. Healing should be rapid and uneventful, with a good solid clot in the socket to protect it and encourage proper healing. Rest and proper nutrition stimulate the healing process, so be sure that you get both. You must be pleased to be rid of that painful, offensive tooth, so that your body can be totally healthy once more. In a few days you will probably have forgotten all about this experience, except when your tongue accidentally goes looking at its new space."

Contrast this matter-of-fact approach with one like the following: "This tooth is really locked into that bone and I'm going to have a hard time removing it. Let's start by trying this way. No, Miss Assistant, not that elevator, I want those other forceps. Hurry up with that suction! This is really a tough one! I won't be surprised if you have trouble after this extraction. You're going to have a mighty sore jaw, and I don't know how much swelling and discoloration you can expect. Get this prescription filled on your way home . . . it's for the pain." Then the postoperative instructions are given: "Since this extraction was so difficult, I'm concerned about development of a dry socket or an infection. If your jaw starts to ache, be sure to call me and get in here at once; don't put it off, for it will only get worse. This will probably have to be treated or packed again, too. I'll see that you get an appointment tomorrow for me to check it."

One can easily see from the foregoing examples that both verbal and non-verbal communication play an extremely important role in the establishment of proper rapport with one's patients. Every attempt should be made to use both forms of communication constructively as means of suggestion. Words and phrases that have negative connotations, whether intentional or inadvertent, should be avoided whenever possible.

RECOGNITION AND MANAGEMENT OF THE ANXIOUS PATIENT

An opportunity to learn about the patient is provided during the initial examination and pretreatment history and physical evaluation. The full significance of the patient's history is best learned through direct questioning and attentive listening. Frequently, the manner in which a particular question is answered is more important than, or even directly contradictory to, the answer that is given. Thus the patient who replies that he is not unduly fearful or nervous, in a tone of voice that belies his statement, is in effect saying that he *is* fearful and concerned.

In addition, patients should not be cut unduly short in their replies to broad queries. Careful listening by the dentist is certain to assist him in the recognition of the anxious patient. By both verbal and nonverbal communication the patient can express resentment, fear, and rejection. The patient who coughs, "has a sinus problem," or cannot get his head adjusted on the headrest is in effect saying, "I know I have to do this, but I don't have to enjoy it; I'll delay it as much as I can." The patient who sits in the chair and wrings his hands or his handkerchief is waiting to be asked what is wrong, so that he can answer. Some children may go even to the extent of vomiting to avoid dental treatment.

It should occur to the dentist to offer help to the woman patient who chatters incessantly to delay her dentistry. The dentist may say: "Mrs. Smith, you seem particularly anxious today, why don't you just relax?" His patient will probably reply, "I can't!" This gives the practitioner an opportunity to demonstrate to her how relaxation can be achieved. This may be done in many ways. Spending a few minutes in teaching now can save much time later. A simple way is to demonstrate the difference in perception between tension and relaxation.

While holding the patient's arm by the wrist, the dentist asks her to relax her hand and to "let it go limp and be completely relaxed." When the hand is relaxed, the point of an explorer is pressed into the back of the hand enough to depress but not penetrate the tissue. Next the patient is instructed to make a very tight fist, and pressure with the explorer is repeated. Obviously the tense fist will feel the sensation more than the relaxed hand. The patient should then be told: "Your entire body was as tense as your fist when you entered the office. Such tension works against your comfort, since it magnifies even the most minimal sensations. If you will practice keeping your entire body relaxed, dentistry will be much more pleasant."

There are numerous ways to determine whether patients are tense or relaxed during their dental work. One need not rely only on signs such as rapid pulse, flushed face, erratic breathing, and elevated blood pressure to know that a patient is anxious. Some patients' eyes and adjacent muscle tissue give indications of their increasing tension; others grasp the armrest; others like the idea of keeping their palms open and turned up in their laps as a reminder to relax. The dentist can train himself to become aware, when he works, of cues he would not normally observe. Every dentist is aware of the patient who tries to avoid dental treatment by lifting his head higher and higher or by turning away from the dentist. Fear and tension are often demonstrated by the patient who holds his breath without realizing it. Once this is pointed out to him, the simple exercise of remembering to breathe gives him something constructive to do to counteract fear.

When emotion is intense, there are widespread changes that take place in every part of the body and affect all of its functions. Nervous and other physiological processes are altered, thoughts and actions are affected, the degree of adjustment is disrupted. The patient must be assisted to overcome fear of physical pain as well as psychological pain. The dentist must remember that there is, in each individual, some need to be dependent, which the practitioner can accept and use constructively in dentistry. To accomplish this means that he must be aware of his patient's needs. This can often be managed most easily through a system of constructive positive suggestion, adapted for each individual dental situation.

One of the first difficulties encountered in the office occurs when radiographs are attempted. The patient either warns the dentist or demonstrates that he is a "gagger." There are a number of responses to this discovery, depending on the severity of the problem and the individual involved. One of the first and simplest approaches is an attempt to alter the physiology. The patient can be told that he will be given some medication that will keep the films from bothering him. Some ordinary table salt, NaCl, is used and about $1/16$ of a teaspoonful is placed on the back of the patient's tongue. It is explained to the patient that this salty substance will dissolve and inhibit the gag reflex so that the radiograph can be taken more easily. With children it is helpful to paint the film with a salty, brightly colored substance such as Merthiolate. In this manner the salty taste acts as a distraction while its placebo effect aids both patient and practitioner through an otherwise annoying procedure.

As every dentist should know, it is physiologically impossible to gag while one is holding his breath. If the patient recognizes that it is necessary to hold his breath for the quarter second the radiograph takes—"so that the film does not move"—two purposes are again accomplished. The dentist obtains the radiograph and the patient does not gag. In similar technique the patient is encouraged to change his breathing pattern, by breathing either through his mouth or nose or by "panting, like a dog."

Although not all of the above examples relate specifically to the control of pain or anxiety, they do emphasize the importance of suggestion, particularly that of a diversionary nature, in assisting the dental patient through a bothersome episode. Additionally, discussion has indicated both the importance and the means of recognizing those individuals who are in need of special attention. Just as the dentist can use both verbal and nonverbal communication to his advantage, the alert clinician will realize that patients also (usually subconsciously) use the same means of communication in asking for assistance. Being cognizant of these aspects places the dentist in a position to both recognize and treat special patients with special techniques.

THE ROLE OF SUGGESTION IN CONSCIOUS-SEDATION

With the rapid increase in the use of conscious-sedation in the dental office, it is now more important than ever that the dentist realize the impact that suggestion may have on his patients. Suggestions can be direct or implied, verbal or nonverbal, positive or negative. In the comfortable, half-asleep, inevitable state of close rapport that exists with conscious-sedation, iatrogenic health becomes a serious consideration. The dentist should have a recognition of the total needs of the patient and an awareness of the emotional and psychological significance of the oral cavity. His suggestions, as well as his manner, should be positive. He may even have to learn new attitudes toward patients.

Every opportunity to employ suggestion to enhance the pharmacological effect of drugs used for the production of conscious-sedation should be used. Prior to the conscious-sedative procedure the patient should be assured that he will not go to sleep but, rather, will be in a relaxed, comfortable, and indifferent state. Depending on the drugs that are to be used, various subjective symptoms the patient is likely to experience should be defined.

The dentist may then take advantage of known pharmacological effects to further enhance the suggestions he is making. For example, inhalation of nitrous oxide and oxygen will produce a tingling sensation in the hands and feet. By stating "Notice how you become calmed and relaxed as your hands and feet begin to tingle" the practitioner is able to enhance the pharmacological effect with the use of suggestion. Similar statements may be made as other agents are administered. In this manner many patients may be placed in a calmed and relaxed state with the use of minimal drug doses.

If the dentist fails to adequately explain the conscious-sedative procedure, many patients may actually require greater drug doses. These fearful patients may really become more fearful as medications are administered and effect realized. Failing to realize that various sensations (tingling, numbness, euphoria, etc.) are normal and to be expected, these persons may feel that "something is wrong" and become more fearful and apprehensive. Patients should be questioned as to sensations they are realizing and then reassured that these are normal and expected (assuming, of course, that this is the case). Psychological patient preparation must not be overlooked for the sake of expediency.

SUGGESTION PLUS CONSCIOUS-SEDATION IN THE ELIMINATION OF ANXIETY

The combination of conscious-sedation plus suggestion may also be used to educate dental patients and to eliminate many inherent but unfounded fears concerning dental treatment. Using the assistance of conscious-sedation, the dentist may make appropriate suggestions that can aid the patient to achieve a greater degree of relaxation and freedom from fear than that produced by pharmacological means alone. Suggestions to the effect that conscious-sedation is being used as an aid for the patient to learn that dentistry need not be physically or psychologically traumatic accompany other suggestions. With the patient in the relaxed conscious-sedative state, suggestions are more likely to be accepted, and teaching the patient to accept dental treatment is easily accomplished in many instances. After the initial conscious-sedation appointment the patient may be congratulated on his excellent performance and a brief statement may be made to the effect that the conscious-sedative experience is being temporarily employed to assist him to overcome fears related to dental treatment.

Subsequent appointments rely to a greater degree on the influence of suggestion than on drug actions to produce the desired effects. The patient may be informed that much less medication is being required, since he is learning to overcome his fears. Once again he is congratulated on his performance and the fine progress that he is making in overcoming dentally related fears through the use of conscious-sedation.

By combining the proper use of suggestion with conscious-sedation many a patient may be "weaned" from a temporary pharmacological crutch provided during his learning experience. In many instances as few as one or two appointments carried out with the aid of conscious-sedation are all that are required to convert a previously anxious and uncooperative dental patient into a relaxed and cooperative one.

Following an appointment in which conscious-sedation has been employed, the patient frequently remarks that "anticipation of the appointment" was out of all proportion to the actual dental procedure. It is not uncommon for patients to state that the dental procedure carried out with the aid of conscious-sedation was actually an enjoyable experience and that apprehension and anxiety prior to the next office visit will be minimal. In effect *the conscious-sedative experience itself was a learning experience.*

Just as one may enhance pharmacological effects through the use of suggestion, the learning experience provided through the aid of conscious-sedation may be enhanced as well. Just as suggestion may be used as an aid in the production of conscious-sedation, conscious-sedation may be used as an aid to the acceptance of suggestions. When this combination is employed, many patients will learn that dentistry is not to be feared and that it can be performed in a comfortable and pain-free manner. After conscious-sedation has been used in the learning process, its use may be discontinued whenever a sufficient degree of patient confidence has been gained and anxiety diminished.

SUMMARY

Advances in dentistry have led to new materials and new techniques in all phases of dental practice. A great deal more is known today about pain perception, pain reaction, and the control of both aspects. The use of local anesthesia combined with conscious-sedation and suggestion to enhance its effectiveness has contributed immeasurably to the control of pain and anxiety in dental patients. It is now both practical and realistic to approach complete dental service with the patient in a conscious, comfortable, and cooperative state. Most dental procedures can be performed more accurately and efficiently if the patient is conscious and responsive to direction. By using the psychological principles of suggestion, with or without pharmacological adjuncts, even the most phobic and anxious dental patients can be managed satisfactorily. In many instances, dental fears and phobias can be eliminated or reduced through the use of conscious-sedation coupled with appropriate use of suggestion. Realization of the importance of verbal and nonverbal communication is an integral part of dental practice. No more than psyche and soma can be separated in consideration of the body and its health can words and actions be separated in their effects on the body and its health.

Chapter 6

INHALATION SEDATION—NITROUS OXIDE AND OXYGEN

The value, safety, and convenience of nitrous oxide in the production of conscious-sedation are appreciated by all who have had experience with this adjunct to the control of operative dental pain and apprehension. Yet today nitrous oxide, the first agent employed for the production of general anesthesia, remains one of the most misunderstood agents used for the production of conscious-sedation.

To a large measure this misunderstanding may be attributed to its association with the production of general anesthesia, particularly the outmoded technique of "secondary saturation." That technique, popular in the early 1900s, relied on hypoxia, produced through administration of 100% nitrous oxide, to render the patient insensitive to the pain of dental surgery. Although the procedure was fraught with danger, a lack of scientific knowledge permitted practitioners of the day to pursue this new-found method of pain control with great vigor. Needless to say, the hazards associated with the hypoxic state were manifested on a great many occasions and use of nitrous oxide fell into disrepute.

Unfortunately, the stigma that became associated with nitrous oxide plus its association with the production of general anesthesia have led the uninformed practitioner of today, who is unaware of the effects of nitrous oxide in subanesthetic doses, to shy away from this agent.

A better understanding of the pharmacology and objectives of nitrous oxide and oxygen sedation has led to the development of conscious-sedative techniques and the production of analgesia machines, resulting in the return of this agent to all areas of dental practice.

Nitrous oxide and oxygen sedation has a definite place in the spectrum of pain control, and it definitely has a place in the pain and apprehension control armamentarium of every dental practitioner.

HISTORY

One year after his discovery of oxygen, Joseph Priestley in 1772 prepared nitrous oxide, but it was not until 1795 that its anesthetic properties were suspected by Sir Humphrey Davy. In 1799 Davy constructed a gas machine and in 1800 described the analgesia produced by nitrous oxide inhalation in relief of pain caused by a wisdom tooth, thus suggesting its possible use as an anesthetic agent.

Horace Wells, the man officially recognized as the discoverer of general anesthesia, was also the first to benefit from his discovery. In 1844 Wells had a painful tooth extracted while under the influence of nitrous oxide. On awakening he proclaimed that "a new era in tooth pulling" had been born.

Edmund A. Andrews in 1868 recognized the effects of pure nitrous oxide as those of asphyxia and suggested that oxygen, in a concentration of at least 20%, be administered with nitrous oxide. Today nitrous oxide remains the most popular primary agent for the production of general anesthesia.

CHEMISTRY

Nitrous oxide, the only inorganic inhalation agent, is a colorless, sweet-smelling gas with a density of 1.5 (air = 1 at 25° C.) and a boiling point of −89.5° C. It is prepared commercially by heating ammonium nitrate crystals in an iron retort at 240° C.

$$NH_4NO_3 \xrightarrow{\text{heat}} N_2O + 2H_2O$$

Impurities produced by manufacture include nitrogen, ammonia, and higher oxide of nitrogen, particularly nitric oxide (NO), which may combine with hemoglobin, as does carbon monoxide.

All impurities of nitrous oxide are removed by a chemical scrubbing process prior to compression at 50-atmosphere pressure to a liquid and storage of the gas at 650 to 800 pounds per square inch (psi) in blue cylinders.

The pressure within the cylinders depends on the gaseous phase and remains constant until all the liquid nitrous oxide has evaporated. It then falls precipitously. Therefore one cannot know the degree of filling of a cylinder after its use, so long as a pressure of 750 psi is registered.

Nitrous oxide is neither explosive nor flammable, but it supports combustion as well as oxygen. The blood/gas solubility coefficient for this gas is 0.47, accounting for the relatively rapid onset and recovery times with this agent.

PHARMACOLOGY

Nitrous oxide, the weakest of all agents, is a 15% potent anesthetic agent and is effective primarily through the replacement of nitrogen in the bloodstream. Its action within the bloodstream is purely physical and it combines chemically with no tissues.

In general, one may characterize the pharmacological effects of nitrous oxide as extremely mild when it is administered with adequate oxygen.

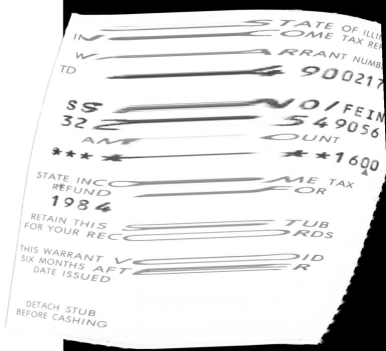

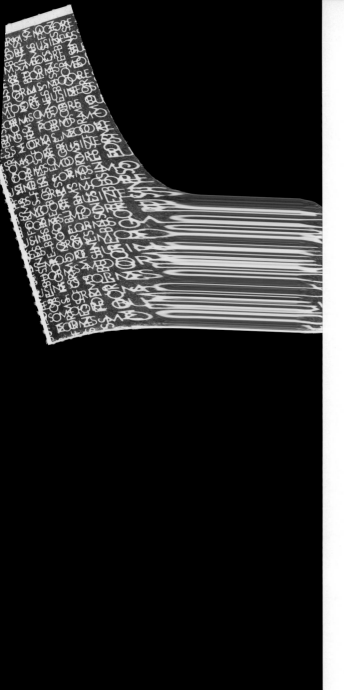

Central nervous system

The primary site of action of nitrous oxide is the central nervous system. In the conscious state a variety of signs and symptoms occur that reflect the effect of nitrous oxide on this system. These are related to the inhaled concentration of the agent. The dentist who has produced conscious-sedation with the use of nitrous oxide is able to appreciate that there is a considerable range of patient response.

The signs and symptoms described here (Table 2) indicate the range of concentrations over which the responses are obtained. Not all individuals will experience the same sensations or exhibit the same objective signs.

Somnolence, or the production of sleep, begins in almost all patients even with very low concentrations of nitrous oxide and increases to general anesthesia as the concentration rises. Dissociation, which includes the inability to accurately perceive one's spatial orientation, reaches its peak effect in the analgesia range.

To some patients dissociation is an unpleasant sensation, not unlike the dysphoric state produced in a few patients by narcotic analgetics. A reduction in the inhaled concentration of nitrous oxide will usually eliminate the unpleasant sensation while maintaining a satisfactory degree of conscious-

Table 2. Signs and symptoms in response to nitrous oxide and oxygen conscious-sedation

Concentration N_2O	Response
10% to 20%	Body warmth
	Tingling of hands and feet
20% to 30%	Circumoral numbness
	Numbness of thighs
20% to 40%	Numbness of tongue
	Numbness of hands and feet
	Droning sounds present
	Hearing distinct but distant
	Dissociation begins and reaches peak
	Mild sleepiness
	Analgesia (maximum at 30%)
	Euphoria
	Feeling of heaviness or lightness of body
30% to 50%	Sweating
	Nausea
	Amnesia
	Increased sleepiness
40% to 60%	Dreaming, laughing, giddiness
	Further increased sleepiness, tending toward unconsciousness
	Increased nausea and vomiting
50% and over	Unconsciousness and light general anesthesia

sedation. Throughout the range of concentrations that will produce conscious-sedation the patient is capable of rational response to verbal command. Indeed, maintenance of verbal contact for monitoring purposes is essential to all degrees of conscious-sedation. Signs that the inhaled concentration of nitrous oxide is too great include sweating, nausea, dreaming, uncoordinated movement, report of unpleasant sensations, sluggish response to verbal command, frequent need to remind the patient to open his mouth, laughing or giddiness, or the report of inability to stay awake. It has been shown that the lower limit of nitrous oxide generally capable of producing unconsciousness and light general anesthesia is about 45%, although some persons may exhibit this response at a lower concentration. There should never be any hesitation on the part of the operator to decrease the concentration if the situation warrants. The optimal concentration for the production of sedation and analgesia in the conscious, cooperative patient has been shown to be 35%. These goals may, on occasion, be reached with lower concentrations; rarely will higher concentrations be required.

Careful examination of Table 2 reveals that as the inhaled concentration of nitrous oxide is increased, desirable effects are quickly produced. As the concentration is further increased, desirability increases until a peak effect is reached. If one increases the concentration at this point, undesirable effects begin to appear and become more pronounced as the concentration is increased still further.

It is imperative that one recognize this effect when administering nitrous oxide lest the patient be exposed to a concentration that exceeds his optimum. Should the patient experience undesirable effects, it is often difficult to convince him that the effect can be reversed and that he can be placed in a comfortable state. By presenting gradually increasing concentrations of nitrous oxide to the patient, the operator is more likely to achieve the maximum desired effect while avoiding unpleasantness.

Cardiovascular system

Responses of the cardiovascular system in the conscious patient to inhalation of nitrous oxide and oxygen have been shown to parallel those of inhaling 100% oxygen. There is an insignificant rise in mean arterial pressure caused by an increase in total peripheral resistance while cardiac output falls, as does the work of the heart.

Nitrous oxide has a relatively low blood/gas solubility coefficient, 0.47. The alveolar concentration of this gas reflects the blood/gas levels and therefore the inhaled concentration rapidly affects the tissue levels of the gas. This means that inhalation of nitrous oxide will be rapidly effective and the termination of its effects equally rapid. The peak effect at a given concentration, as well as return to the presedation state, will be achieved in 3 to 5 minutes.

Nitrous oxide does not combine with any formed elements of the blood, being carried strictly in physical solution. It is fifteen times as soluble in blood as the nitrogen that it replaces.

Respiratory system

As with the cardiovascular system, the effects of nitrous oxide when administered with adequate amounts of oxygen are negligible on this system. However, it has been observed to increase the respiratory minute volume without depressing the response of the respiratory center to carbon dioxide administration.

Transport across the pulmonary epithelium accounts for the uptake and excretion of the vast majority of nitrous oxide in the body. The drug is primarily eliminated unchanged by the lungs, with an insignificant amount being excreted unchanged through the skin.

Other organs and systems

Although several systems have been demonstrated to be adversely affected by prolonged exposure to nitrous oxide at high concentrations, these findings are of little, if any, clinical significance. Nitrous oxide, when administered with adequate oxygen (at least 20% in the inspired air), may be considered to be inert and nontoxic. It produces little if any effect on any system other than the central nervous system. The production of surgical anesthesia or tissue damage by this agent must be considered to be caused by hypoxia that accompanied its administration.

Presently various groups are examining the effects of trace amounts of nitrous oxide on operating room personnel as well as dentists and their auxiliaries who are chronically exposed to this agent. Implications have been made that trace amounts of nitrous oxide contribute to an increase in the spontaneous abortion rate as well as the initiation of various pathological states. Some authors recommend the use of scavenging devices, laminar flow air circulating units, or other methods of keeping nitrous oxide concentrations in the operating room below 50 parts per million. As yet, no convincing studies exist to document the danger of trace amounts of nitrous oxide. Undoubtedly in the future studies that either confirm or deny these implications will appear, as well as government regulations aimed at controlling the administration of this agent should it be proved hazardous.

CLINICAL CONSIDERATIONS

If one is to employ nitrous oxide and oxygen for the production of conscious-sedation, he must bear in mind the fact that the primary objective is to provide the patient with a feeling of pleasant relaxation. Although nitrous oxide is capable of producing both analgesia and amnesia, these are fringe benefits to be gained and not objectives to be sought.

Patient selection

The success of nitrous oxide for the production of conscious-sedation depends on a thorough understanding of the pharmacology of the agent, its abilities and its limitations, as well as on proper patient selection and preparation.

Patient selection is based on the information gained during the pretreatment history and physical evaluation. Both the physical and psychological needs of the patient must be taken into consideration. As a general rule one may say that the poorer the patient's physical condition the greater the need for conscious-sedation. A patient who is in poor health is less able to tolerate the physical stresses placed on him by a long, trying, or uncomfortable dental appointment.

Whether conscious-sedation should be employed with the use of nitrous oxide or with other, more potent drugs administered via parenteral routes may be determined by examining the patient's psychological condition. His "level of awareness" must be determined by attentive listening to replies during history taking while carefully observing the patient for signs of dentally related psychological distress. Awareness of previous unpleasant dental experiences the patient may have had is also important.

In contrast to this concept—the poorer the physical condition, the greater the indication for conscious-sedation—there is another—the poorer the psychological condition, the less the indication for nitrous oxide sedation. Since this drug is the weakest agent available, it is only useful for calming those patients who may be considered to be mildly apprehensive. Patients who are judged to be moderately or very apprehensive will require the use of more potent drugs or drug combinations.

This is not to say that nitrous oxide sedation is of little value in treating apprehensive patients. To the contrary, a great many patients who now avoid dental treatment or who suffer through the appointment while considering the visit one of life's necessary evils may be satisfactorily managed with the use of nitrous oxide sedation.

However, the dentist must develop the skills necessary to properly select that group of patients in which this means of apprehension control is most likely to be successful. Attempting to manage all patients with this modality is sure to lead to many unsuccessful results and eventual disenchantment with the technique.

Patient preparation—psychological

After the prospective candidate for nitrous oxide sedation has been selected, a certain amount of psychological preparation is desirable. The first order of business is to briefly and concisely explain the philosophy of conscious-sedation, using words the layman is sure to understand. He must be told that the medication that will be administered will not "put him to sleep."

He must be assured that he will be fully aware of his surroundings and in full control of his faculties at all times, yet be calmed and relaxed and have an indifferent attitude toward the dental treatment.

The subjective symptoms he will experience while under the influence of nitrous oxide should be described. Here the role of suggestion becomes a very definite part of the conscious-sedative technique. Taking advantage of known pharmacological properties of nitrous oxide lets its effect be enhanced through the use of appropriate suggestions.

The patient should be familiarized with the nasal mask and told that he will be able to control the degree of sedation he will experience, by breathing through his nose for a greater effect or through his mouth for a lessened effect. If the patient is made to realize that the ability to control the sedative effect rests with him, he is less likely to be fearful or hesitant to experience conscious-sedation, a technique that may be new to him. In addition, he is less prone to associate inhalation sedation with a previous general anesthetic experience, which may have been unpleasant.

After having psychologically prepared the patient for nitrous oxide sedation at an introductory appointment (during which few if any dental procedures are to be performed), one may choose to seat the patient in the dental chair and "allow" him to briefly sample the sedative experience. In this manner the patient's first exposure to nitrous oxide sedation comes at a time when apprehension is at a low ebb. The initial experience, therefore, is more likely to be favorable, thus building confidence in both the technique and the operator. This initial exposure should be very brief. One is attempting not only to introduce the patient to the state of pleasant relaxation that can be produced but also to whet the appetite for future trials.

For introducing a child to nitrous oxide sedation the approach is not unlike the introduction used for an adult except that the dentist must be certain that his presentation is unhurried and does not give the impression of being forceful. A careful selection of descriptive words and phrases commensurate with the child's intellectual level will aid in the presentation. Reference to fantasy-world heroes, space travel, fairyland gardens, etc. may be accompanied by spraying the nasal mask with scented alcohol prior to "allowing" the child to enter a mystical world by inhaling the "magical" scents.

Patient preparation—physical

A minimum amount of patient preparation from a physical standpoint is also required prior to the use of nitrous oxide sedation.

A suggestion should be made to the patient that he wear loose-fitting, comfortable garments the day of the dental appointment, since one is much more able to relax if he is not confined by tight, restricting shirt collars and the like. The patient should also be given instructions regarding food intake prior to the appointment. He should be told that the meal eaten prior to the office visit should be consumed about 2 to 3 hours before the scheduled appointment and should consist of light liquids such as broth, tea, gelatin, etc.

Since the patient will be conscious throughout the procedure, the presence of food in the stomach is not dangerous, as it is with unconscious techniques. However, by his eating the prescribed meal the patient's caloric needs are met while the liquids are quickly absorbed from the stomach. In this manner, the patient arrives at the office with an essentially empty stomach, which precludes almost entirely the possibility of vomiting—an episode that, while not hazardous, is unpleasant at best. Patients should also be cautioned not to fast prior to the visit. Fasting may lead to a mild hypoglycemic state that may contribute to nausea.

My experience with patients who have followed the restrictions governing presedative food intake has been quite favorable. Only on rare occasions have any patients become nauseated, and retching or vomiting has not been encountered in the properly prepared patient.

TECHNICAL APPROACH

After all equipment has been checked, to be certain it is in proper working order, the analgesia machine is turned "on" and the breathing bag is filled with 100% oxygen either by adjusting the flowmeter to deliver high flows or by rapidly filling the bag with the flush valve. One should avoid using the flush valve to fill the bag after the nasal mask is in position on the patient's face. The sudden burst of oxygen coupled with the sound of the rapidly flowing gas is certain to startle most patients.

It is important to make sure that the breathing bag is properly filled with oxygen or that the air dilution valve is open when the mask is positioned on the patient's face. If such is not the case, the patient's first breath will collapse the bag, resulting in a sudden inability to breathe and a suffocating sensation to the patient.

Once the mask has been positioned (Fig. 6-1, *A*), the patient is allowed to adjust it to a comfortable position (Fig. 6-1, *B*). This maneuver aids the patient in realizing that he has control of the situation and is in no way being confined or restrained by the apparatus. The nasal mask in position, the operator tightens the adjustment on the breathing tubes that encircle the patient's head and the headrest of the dental chair (Fig. 6-1, *C*). The mask should now be comfortably snug on the patient's face.

At this point the exhalation valve on the mask should be wide open while the air dilution valve is turned to the closed position. One hundred percent oxygen should be flowing into the system at a sufficient flow rate to keep the breathing bag from collapsing on inspiration. A flow of about 5 liters per minute will usually suffice. The patient is instructed to breathe first through his nose and then through his mouth, to demonstrate how he is able to control the degree of effect he will shortly be experiencing.

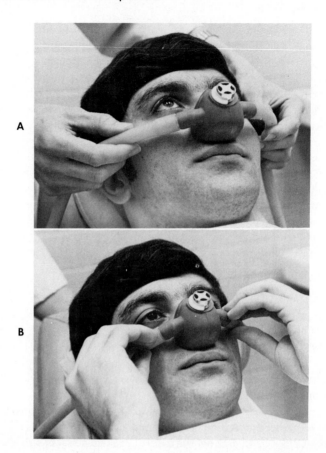

Fig. 6-1. A, Nasal mask positioned on face of patient. **B,** Patient adjusts mask to comfortable position. **C,** Operator secures mask in position by adjusting breathing tubes, which encircle patient's head and headrest of dental chair.

The patient is now ready to begin to inhale the nitrous oxide and oxygen mixture. The oxygen flow is then adjusted to its minimum, usually 3 to 4 liters per minute, while the nitrous oxide flowmeter is adjusted to deliver 0.5 to 1 liter per minute. (See Chapter 7 regarding minimum oxygen flow.)

The patient is told that soon he *may* be noticing the pleasant smell of the nitrous oxide and that he *may* be starting to experience the symptoms previously described.

With the introduction of the word "may," the role of suggestion enters the conscious-sedative technique, and the full measure of its importance should be realized. The operator should take advantage of the known pharmacological properties of nitrous oxide to predict and suggest to the patient how he will be

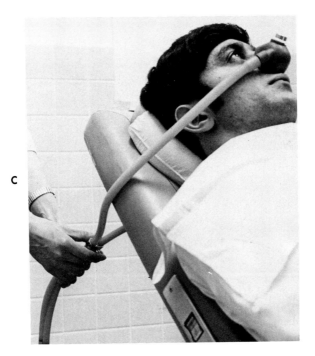

Fig. 6-1, cont'd. For legend see opposite page.

feeling. In this manner the patient gains more confidence in both operator and technique.

As mentioned earlier, not all patients experience the same symptoms, and the dose range over which any given sensation is produced is quite variable. Therefore, care must be taken by the dentist when using the words "may" or "will." For those sensations that are rather variable from patient to patient the word "may" should be stressed. For sensations that are rather predictable in all individuals the word "will" should be employed. Not every patient is able to smell nitrous oxide or experience any noticeable effects at very low concentrations. Hence, he is told what he *may* notice.

Gradually, in stepwise fashion, the nitrous oxide concentration is increased while suggestions are made and questions are asked of the patient in order to determine the degree of sedation being produced and symptoms being experienced. In this way the amount of nitrous oxide being delivered to the patient is slowly increased until a state of pleasant relaxation is produced.

As the concentration is increased, suggestions relevant to the symptoms most often realized at that concentration are made. For example, when the patient is inhaling 30% nitrous oxide, he is told that his hands and feet *will* begin to tingle, he *will probably* notice a numb sensation around his mouth, he *will*

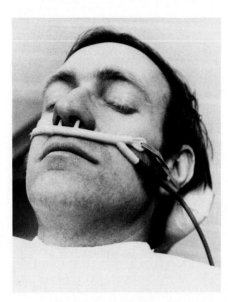

Fig. 6-2. Nasal cannula in position.

feel calmed and relaxed, he *may* feel warm and *may* notice a humming or droning noise, and that his body *may* feel light, as if it is floating, suspended in air, or it *may* feel heavy, as though his limbs are made of lead.

Verbal contact must be maintained with the patient both to enable the dentist to observe his state of consciousness and to determine the subjective symptoms the patient is experiencing. On occasion he should be assured that the sensations noticed are normal (assuming this is the case) and that the procedure is progressing as expected.

Throughout the course of the conscious-sedative procedure the properly prepared and medicated patient will be observed to be sitting calmly relaxed in the dental chair. His mouth will remain open although he continues to breathe through his nose. His eyes will usually be closed. When dentistry is not being performed, a peaceful smile may appear on his face.

Patient monitoring

Although the inherent safety of maintaining the patient in a conscious state precludes significant deviations in vital signs and eliminates the necessity for their continual monitoring, a certain amount of attention must be directed toward monitoring the patient under conscious-sedation.

It is my contention that conscious-sedation, regardless of the drugs employed or route of administration involved, is in no way related to the signs and stages of anesthesia as described by Guedel in 1920. Numerous investigations (Thomas, Pantalone, Buchanan, and Zeedick) have shown that those signs and stages are valid only if one is employing ether anesthesia.

It is unfortunate that Guedel's first stage of ether anesthesia, which he termed the analgesia stage, is frequently and erroneously confused with nitrous oxide conscious-sedation. Through various misnomers (for example, nitrous oxide analgesia) the implication is made that conscious-sedation is in reality a form of general anesthesia or that it is being used for the control of operative pain or that regional analgesia need not accompany it. *Such is not the case.*

Furthermore, a thorough understanding of conscious-sedation and the drugs used to produce it will demonstrate that they have no appreciable effect on any organ or system except the central nervous system. There the effect is to produce an altered state of awareness, and under no ordinary circumstance is the effect great enough to affect regulation of vital functions.

Therefore it is apparent that it is sheer folly to attempt to define the "depth" or the "signs and stages" of a technique that fails to render a patient unconscious or produce changes in vital functions, since these are the only parameters that may be of use in describing a mythical concept, depth of sedation.

On occasion one hears reference to such phrases as "total analgesia" or "the excitement stage." The reader must be assured that total analgesia, or the lack of ability to appreciate *all* degrees of painful stimulation *in the conscious state,* it not possible with pharmacological agents currently available.

Caution must be exercised when conscious-sedation is being employed lest the uninitiated to led to believe that operative pain can be controlled in the conscious patient by increasing the dose of the sedative drug. Only through the production of unconsciousness is it possible to eliminate all degrees of operative pain in the absence of regional analgesia.

It is my belief that the phrase "excitement stage" as well as the use of ether anesthesia should be stricken from medical and dental practice. Anyone who has ever received an ether anesthetic will agree that its use is a cruel and inhumane method for the production of general anesthesia, as compared to present-day techniques. The phrase "excitement stage," which may rightfully be applied to only the second stage of ether anesthesia, has absolutely *no place* in the terminology describing nitrous oxide conscious-sedation.

The true "excitement stage" can be produced only by ether anesthesia and occurs only after the patient has been rendered unconscious by the drug. Anyone who has had experience with ether anesthesia realizes that the occasional laughing and giddiness produced by nitrous oxide is a far cry from the excitement stage that is seen routinely when ether is employed.

Some common misconceptions concerning conscious-sedation having been dispelled, a brief description of monitoring procedures is in order. All patients undergoing conscious-sedation should be observed throughout the procedure for the presence of three parameters: (1) consciousness, (2) comfort, and (3) cooperation.

Consciousness. It is imperative that the patient remain conscious at all times, regardless of the drug or route of administration chosen for the conscious-sedative technique. Verbal contact has been shown to be the best means of monitoring the patient for his state of consciousness. When nitrous oxide is employed for sedation, the patient should not be encouraged to talk frequently. Speaking tends to encourage mouth breathing and a subsequent decrease in drug effect. Intermittent periods of mouth and nasal breathing result in a waxing and waning of effect rather than maintenance of a constant effect. Appropriate response to the verbal commands (open or close your mouth, etc.) that ordinarily accompany dental procedures will suffice in establishing verbal contact. *All patients* must be capable of rational response to command at *all times*. With the presence of consciousness comes stability of vital functions, and there are only insignificant deviations in vital signs.

Comfort. Certainly one of the main objectives of conscious-sedation is the production of a state in which the patient is relaxed and comfortable. This state will usually be achieved with nitrous oxide in concentration of about 30% to 35%. Although the patient remains conscious, concentrations greater than this are likely to result in discomfort from intensity of effect or dysphoric sensations. A few patients may experience nausea. Patient comfort can be assessed while maintaining verbal contact. Once an initial state of pleasant relaxation is established, the patient should be informed that this state will be maintained throughout the appointment. If at any time the effect becomes uncomfortably intense, he may take a few breaths through his mouth. On noticing the presence of mouth breathing, the dentist may readjust the nitrous oxide concentration to a lower level. Frequent deep breaths by the patient through his nose should indicate to the dentist a need for readjustment of nitrous oxide concentrations to higher levels. It is imperative that the dose administered be one that places the patient in a comfortable as well as a conscious state.

Cooperation. One of the primary benefits to the *dentist* to be gained from conscious-sedation is patient cooperation. Most patients who are properly selected and prepared will exhibit the greatest degree of cooperation while inhaling nitrous oxide in concentrations between 30% and 35%.

Patients remaining uncooperative at concentrations below that range may become cooperative as the concentration is increased. A few patients will require concentrations greater than 35%. Those patients failing to become cooperative at concentrations greater than 35% and less than 50% should be considered candidates for another form of conscious-sedation (for example, an intravenous conscious-sedative technique).

Concentration of nitrous oxide

The concentration of nitrous oxide necessary for the production of conscious-sedation will vary from 15% to 50%, depending on the level of awareness of each patient and how he is affected by the agent. As a result the concentration of nitrous oxide may be slowly increased until the patient feels pleasantly relaxed while fulfilling all requirements necessary for the safe conduct of conscious-sedation. The concentration of nitrous oxide should be decreased if the patient does any of the following:

1. Spontaneously begins to breathe through his mouth
2. States that the effects of the agent are uncomfortable, too intense, etc.
3. Complains of nausea
4. Talks incoherently or relates the presence of dreams
5. Fails to respond rationally or responds sluggishly to verbal command
6. States that he is about to "fall asleep"
7. Makes uncoordinated movements
8. Begins to perspire
9. Must be frequently reminded to open his mouth
10. Becomes uncooperative
11. Laughs, cries, or becomes giddy

If any of the above signs or symptoms occurs, the inhaled concentration of nitrous oxide should be readjusted to once again place the patient in the proper state. As a general rule, should the patient exhibit any of the preceding signs or experience symptoms that are unpleasant, the concentration of nitrous oxide is too great and should be reduced. After having successfully adjusted the concentration to the proper level for that patient, the dentist should see that a note to that effect is made a part of the patient's permanent record. Reference to the proper concentration and adjustment of the flowmeters appropriately will facilitate the production of conscious-sedation at future appointments.

Regional analgesia

After having placed the patient under the effects of conscious-sedation at the proper dosage level, the dentist may now proceed to apply the regional analgesic techniques that are required for the control of operative pain. The patient who was previously fearful and apprehensive about a procedure will now accept it willingly, his mood having been sufficiently altered by the medication. In addition, the degree of analgesia provided by the agent will render the patient less sensitive to any minor discomfort that may be associated with needle insertion.

All but the most innocuous dental procedures must be accompanied by the use of regional analgesia. This is not to say that all procedures require the use of regional analgesia. Routine dentistry involves many minor procedures that, although annoying to the patient, are not particularly painful. Such procedures as an oral examination, the polishing of a restoration, or the taking of a radiograph might be more easily accomplished with the aid of nitrous oxide sedation.

Control of the gag response, which is largely psychological in origin, can be easily accomplished with the use of nitrous oxide sedation. With alteration of the patient's mood and thus a decrease in psychological influence, procedures that were previously impossible or difficult at best are frequently accomplished with ease.

Termination of procedure

After the dental procedure has been satisfactorily completed through the use of conscious-sedation, the flow of nitrous oxide is discontinued and the patient allowed to breathe 100% oxygen for several minutes.

Although it is difficult to conceive of this phenomenon occurring in a relatively healthy patient following brief exposure to low doses of nitrous oxide, administration of pure oxygen at the completion of the procedure will preclude entirely the possibility of diffusion hypoxia.

Diffusion hypoxia occurs when the inhalation of nitrous oxide is discontinued and the patient is allowed to breathe room air. As a result of rapid elimination of nitrous oxide from the blood the alveolar oxygen concentration is diluted, resulting in a brief period of hypoxia. I do not consider this phenomenon to be of any clinical importance following conscious-sedation.

Within 5 to 10 minutes the patient is usually in satisfactory condition for dismissal from the office. Rapid elimination of nitrous oxide from the body makes it unnecessary for the patient to be detained or escorted from the office unless in the dentist's opinion the patient has any residual effects that make dismissal unwise.

Contraindications to nitrous oxide and oxygen conscious-sedation

Conscious-sedation with the use of nitrous oxide and oxygen is contraindicated in those patients with whom communication is difficult. Such patients may include the very young child or the mentally retarded individual. Since a degree of patient preparation and cooperation is required with this agent, its use would be impossible under these circumstances in most instances.

Since the gas in inhaled through the nostrils, nasal obstruction from any cause, if severe enough to prevent easy inhalation, is an absolute contraindication to its use. I do not believe that pregnancy, asthma, epilepsy, or psychiatric disorder per se contraindicates the use of nitrous oxide sedation.

From a medicolegal aspect one tries to avoid performing elective dental services on women who are in their first trimester of pregnancy. However, should emergency dental care be necessary during this period, the patient will fare better if stress and apprehension are eliminated through the use of nitrous oxide sedation. There is no human indication of teratogenic effects of nitrous oxide.

Patients suffering from asthma or epilepsy are particularly good candidates for the use of conscious-sedation. In many patients the attacks of either asthma or epilepsy are provoked by emotionally trying episodes. Control of emotional stress through the use of conscious-sedation will allow those individuals to better tolerate the dental environment.

In patients who are under psychiatric care the use of conscious-sedation with nitrous oxide or any other drug is not contraindicated. These patients frequently present behavioral and/or psychological problems that make the rendering of dental services impossible without the aid of conscious-sedation. With the use of sedative techniques, however, many of these problem patients may satisfactorily undergo dental treatment without resort to general anesthesia being necessary. One must bear in mind, however, that many of these patients are taking medications to control their disorder. Having knowledge of the drug and its pharmacology is important before proceeding with the sedative procedure. In many instances a reduction in the dose of the sedative agent is required.

SUMMARY

The principles and techniques of conscious-sedation through the use of nitrous oxide and oxygen are presented. Pertinent aspects of the chemistry, pharmacology, physiology, subjective symptoms, and objective signs of nitrous oxide and oxygen inhalation are discussed as they apply to the conscious patient. The importance of patient selection and preparation and the role of suggestion are stressed.

Chapter 7

INHALATION SEDATION EQUIPMENT

The dentist employing nitrous oxide and oxygen for the production of conscious-sedation must have a thorough knowledge of the equipment he is using, as well as an understanding of the agents he is delivering and their effects upon the patient. It is important that all items be in proper order and functioning correctly at all times if the success and safety of the sedative technique are to be assured.

ANALGESIA MACHINES

Although many different pieces of equipment are available from which one may choose, all have certain basic components in common. Variations that exist allow one to select the setup best suited to the personal requirements of expense, convenience, durability, etc. The components held in common by all analgesia machines are discussed here.

Gas source

The supply of nitrous oxide and oxygen may be derived from one of two sources—a portable or a central system.

Portable gas supply. The cylinders most easily adapted to a portable analgesia machine are size "E." These cylinders contain 420 and 165 gallons of nitrous oxide and oxygen, respectively. Empty, they weigh 15 pounds and are portable to the extent that, once affixed to the analgesia machine, they can be wheeled from one area to another.

To eliminate the possibility of wrong gases being used or wrong cylinders being inadvertently substituted for correct cylinders, the Compressed Gas Association, in cooperation with the American Society of Anesthesiologists and the American Hospital Association, has devised a Pin-index Safety System. This system is based on the matching of pins on the machine with corresponding holes on the outlet of the cylinder and is aimed at the prevention of erroneous interchange of gases. (See Fig. 7-1.)

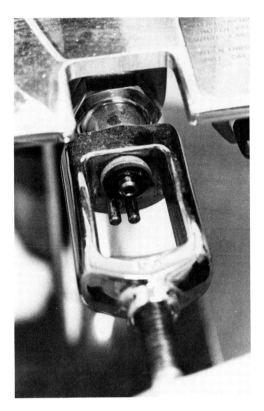

Fig. 7-1. Pin-index Safety System on analgesia machine.

Although this type of gas source is inexpensive in the initial investment, its presence on the analgesia machine makes the machine cumbersome in many operatories, and the frequent replacement of empty cylinders that is required becomes rather bothersome. In addition, using small cylinders as a gas source is expensive to operate when compared to use of the more economical central gas supply.

Central gas supply. The central gas supply system uses large cylinders that contain 3,655 and 1,400 gallons of nitrous oxide (size "H") and oxygen (size "G"), respectively. They are 55 inches tall and weigh 100 pounds when empty.

When this system is employed, the cylinders will usually be located at some distance from the operatory and in an area of easy access. Multiple tanks of nitrous oxide and of oxygen, each having a pressure-reducing regulator affixed, will be attached to their respective manifold systems, each of which in turn is connected with copper tubing to an outlet station in the operatory (Fig. 7-2).

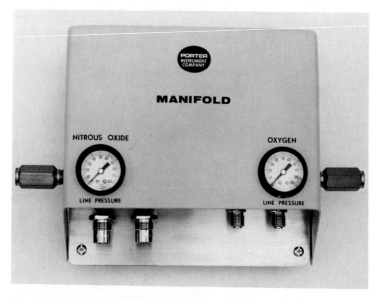

Fig. 7-2. Central nitrous oxide and oxygen manifold system. (Courtesy Porter Instrument Company, Inc.)

Each manifold consists of two cylinder banks—one a service and the other a reserve unit. In this manner one bank of cylinders can be in use at all times, while a reserve bank is ready to be switched on automatically when the service bank empties.

The manifold is equipped with pressure gauges that indicate line pressures (Fig. 7-3). Tank pressure is indicated on the regulator affixed to each cylinder. Optional alarm systems are also available, which may be desk (Fig. 7-4) or wall-mounted (Fig. 7-5) in the dental office to keep personnel advised of gas supplies and thus eliminate the need for frequent inspection of the cylinder area.

The outlet station, located in the operatory, serves as a ready source of gases once the analgesia machine is connected to its appropriate site (Fig. 7-6). Both the outlet station and the gas lines of the machine are Pin-indexed to preclude the possibility of an inadvertent wrong connection. The central gas supply system is equipped with a Diameter Index Safety System that makes it impossible for fittings carrying medical gases to be inappropriately connected.

A less convenient regulator system may also be employed when using large cylinders. With this system a regulator that measures cylinder pressure and reduces the line pressure to about 50 psi is attached to the top of each cylinder. Although less expensive to install than the manifold system, the cylinders must be turned on and off manually each day and will not switch from service

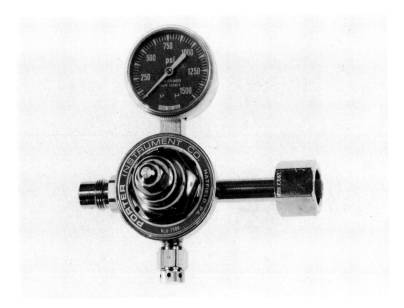

Fig. 7-3. Regulator for large cylinders. (Courtesy Porter Instrument Company, Inc.)

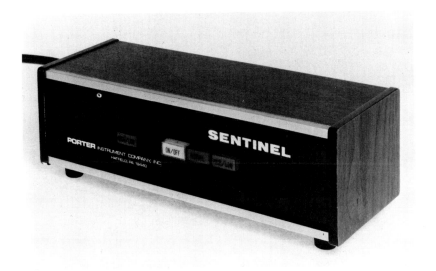

Fig. 7-4. Desk model alarm system. (Courtesy Porter Instrument Company, Inc.)

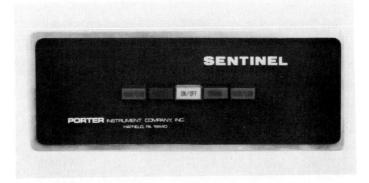

Fig. 7-5. Wall-mounted alarm system. (Courtesy Porter Instrument Company, Inc.)

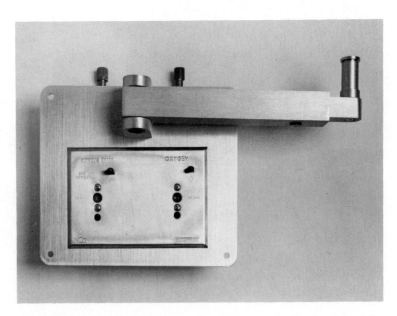

Fig. 7-6. Pin-indexed outlet station with telescoping mounting bracket for attachment of analgesia machine. (Courtesy Porter Instrument Company, Inc.)

to reserve cylinders automatically. If desired, flexible tubing rather than copper tubing may be used and attached directly to the analgesia machine, rather than through a wall outlet.

Factors common to central and portable systems

Regardless of which gas source is used or the size of the cylinder, certain factors are common to both systems. (1) Nitrous oxide is supplied in blue cylinders at a pressure of about 750 pounds per square inch. This pressure will be registered on the pressure gauge of the regulator or on the machine in a portable system (Fig. 7-7). Within the cylinder nitrous oxide is present as both a liquid and a gas, with the pressure reflected being that of the gaseous phase. As the tank is evacuated, the pressure will remain at the original level until all liquid has been converted to gas. Only then will the pressure decrease as the cylinder is emptied further. Flexible tubing, dials, and flowmeters that regulate the delivery of nitrous oxide are also color-coded blue. (2) Oxygen is supplied in green cylinders at a pressure of about 2,100 pounds per square inch. Unlike nitrous oxide, however, oxygen is present in the cylinder in the gaseous state only. For this reason the pressure of the gas falls in direct proportion to the gas consumed. Flexible tubing, dials, and flowmeters that regulate the delivery of oxygen are also color-coded green. (3) Neither nitrous oxide nor oxygen is explosive or flammable. However, each supports combustion, and they do this equally well. For maximum safety, installation of a central gas supply system for the use of nitrous oxide and oxygen should follow the accepted practices recommended by the National Fire Protection Association and the Compressed Gas Association.

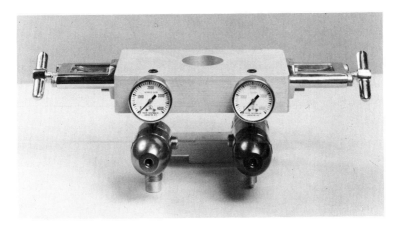

Fig. 7-7. Nitrous oxide and oxygen regulators that affix to portable analgesia machine. Pressure gauges indicate pressure of the gas contained in cylinders. (Courtesy Fraser Sweatman, Inc.)

Recommended safe practices for handling and using medical gases

Following are recommended safety procedures for the handling and use of medical gases.

1. Never permit oil, grease, or other readily combustible substance to come in contact with cylinders, valves, regulators, gauges, hoses, and fittings. Oil and certain gases such as nitrous oxide or oxygen may combine with explosive violence.
2. Do not handle cylinders or apparatus with oily hands or gloves.
3. Prevent sparks or flame from any source from coming in contact with cylinders or equipment.
4. Fully open the cylinder valve when the cylinder is in use.
5. Before placing cylinders in service any paper wrappings should be removed so that cylinder color and label are clearly visible.
6. Do not deface or remove any markings which are used for identification of contents of cylinders.
7. No part of any cylinder containing compressed gas should ever be subjected to temperature above 125° F. A direct flame should never be permitted to come in contact with any part of a compressed gas cylinder.
8. Never tamper with the safety devices in valves or cylinders.
9. Never attempt to repair or alter cylinders.
10. Cylinder valves should be closed at all times except when gas is actually being used or when cylinder is attached to a manifold.
11. Cylinders should be repainted only by the supplier.

Moving cylinders

1. Where caps are provided for valve protection, such caps should be kept on cylinders when cylinders are moved.
2. Never drop cylinders or permit them to strike each other violently.
3. Avoid dragging or sliding cylinders. It is safer to move large cylinders even short distances by using a suitable truck, making sure that the cylinder-retaining strap or chain is fastened in place.

Storing cylinders

1. Cylinders should be stored in a definitely assigned location.
2. Full and empty cylinders should be stored separately, with the storage layout so planned that cylinders comprising old stock can be removed first with a minimum of handling of other cylinders.
3. Storage rooms should be dry, cool, and well ventilated. Where practical, storage rooms should be fireproof.
4. Cylinders should be protected against excessive rise of temperature. Do not store cylinders near radiators or other sources of radiant heat. Do not store cylinders near highly flammable substances such as oil, gasoline, waste, etc.
5. Large cylinders should be placed against a wall to offer some protection against being knocked over. The best practice is to provide a means for a chain fastening large cylinders to the wall.
6. Cylinders may be stored in the open but in such cases should be protected against extremes of weather and from the ground beneath to prevent rusting. During winter, cylinders stored in the open should be protected against

accumulation of ice or snow. In summer, cylinders stored in the open should be screened against continuous direct rays of the sun.

7. Cylinders should not be exposed to continuous dampness and should not be stored near corrosive chemicals or fumes. Rusting will damage the cylinders and may cause the valve protection caps to stick.

8. Cylinders should be protected against tampering by unauthorized individuals.

Withdrawing cylinder contents

1. Never attempt to use contents of a cylinder without a suitable pressure-regulating device. The regulator reduces tank pressure to a line pressure of about 50 pounds per square inch. This provides a uniform flow as cylinder pressure drops and prevents damage to flowmeters by gases at high pressure.

2. After removing valve protection caps, slightly open valve to clear opening of possible dirt and dust.

3. When opening valve, point the outlet away from you. Never use wrenches or tools except those provided or approved by the gas supplier. Never hammer the valve wheel in attempting to open or close the valve.

4. It is important to make sure that the threads on regulators or other auxiliary equipment are the same as those on cylinder valve outlets. Never force connections that do not fit.

5. Never permit gas to enter the regulating device suddenly. Open the cylinder valve slowly.

6. Before regulating device is removed from a cylinder, close the cylinder valve and release all pressure from the device.

7. Always close valves in empty cylinders.*

Control valves

All machines are equipped with control valves having fine adjustments to regulate the flow of gases (Figs. 7-8 and 7-9). It is through these valves that the operator adjusts the total flow and the percentage of each gas being delivered to the patient.

Meters

Meters (flowmeters) are used to indicate the flow of each gas, usually in liters per minute, being delivered by the machine to the patient (Figs. 7-8 and 7-9). This flow is regulated by means of the control valves.

With most analgesia machines one must perform a simple mathematical computation to determine the percentage of each gas being delivered by the machine. The formula for this calculation is as follows:

$$\frac{\text{Gas in question (liters per minute)}}{\text{Total gas flow (liters per minute)}}$$

For example, calculate as follows the percentage of N_2O being delivered if

---

*Adapted from Safe handling of compressed gases, a pamphlet prepared by the Compressed Gas Association.

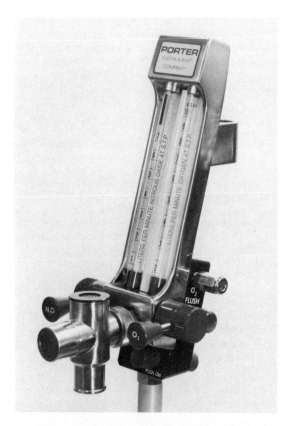

Fig. 7-8. Porter Instrument analgesia machine having levers to control gas flows. (Courtesy Porter Instrument Company, Inc.)

the N_2O flow rate is 2 liters per minute and the O_2 flow rate is 4 liters per minute:

$$\frac{2 \text{ liters } N_2O \text{ per minute}}{2 \text{ liters } N_2O + 4 \text{ liters } O_2 \text{ per minute}} = \frac{2}{6} = \frac{1}{3} = 33^{1}/_{3}\% \; N_2O$$

The remaining $66^{2}/_{3}\%$ is O_2.

One machine currently available, the Quantiflex M.D.M, manufactured by Fraser-Sweatman, Inc. (Fig 7-10), has a feature that eliminates the need for any mathematical computation. The feature on this machine allows one to dial a desired concentration of oxygen and then adjust the total gas flow with another dial. The machine automatically maintains the desired concentration of nitrous oxide while total flow adjustments are made. Should one desire to change the inhaled concentration of nitrous oxide, the machine automatically

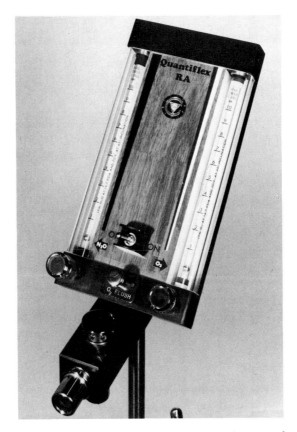

Fig. 7-9. Fraser Sweatman analgesia machine having dials to regulate gas flows. (Courtesy Fraser Sweatman, Inc.)

adjusts the flow of nitrous oxide and oxygen proportionally to deliver the desired concentration while maintaining constant gas flows.

Tubing and mixers

The tubing is used to link the control valves and flowmeters to a common mixing chamber and then to the outflow tube of the machine.

Emergency air valve

Several analgesia machines currently available have emergency air valves attached to the outflow T piece of the unit just above the location for attachment of the reservoir bag (Fig. 7-11). This valve automatically opens, allowing the patient to breathe room air if the gas flow from the machine is inadequate or is interrupted for any reason. For example, should the reservoir bag collapse

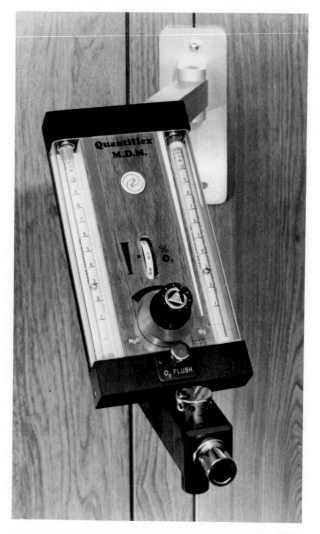

Fig. 7-10. Wall-mounted Quantiflex M.D.M. analgesia machine. (Courtesy Fraser Sweatman, Inc.)

during inhalation because the total gas flow is insufficient to meet the needs of the patient, the valve would open at about −3 cm. of water pressure. When inhaling from a machine that does not possess this valve, many patients experience a suffocating sensation or difficult inhalation as they attempt to inhale from a reservoir bag that collapses during each inspiratory attempt.

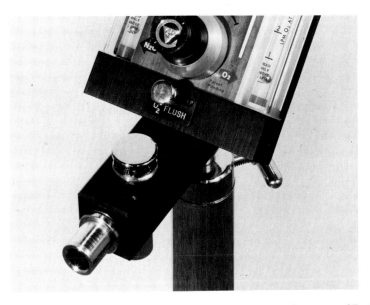

Fig. 7-11. Quantiflex analgesia machine showing emergency air valve on top of T piece of unit. (Courtesy Fraser Sweatman, Inc.)

Check valve

Many manufacturers of analgesia machines are incorporating check valves into the outflow tube. This one-way valve allows the patient to inhale from the reservoir bag while preventing exhalation into it. All exhaled gases must pass from the machine, thus creating a totally nonrebreathing system. The primary advantage of this system is the prevention of carbon dioxide accumulation within the reservoir bag or breathing tubes. The valve is located within the outflow T piece at the point of attachment of the corrugated breathing tube (Fig. 7-11).

Inhaler assembly

The inhaler assembly is usually made of soft rubber and is used to deliver the gas mixture to the patient via his respiratory tract. It is composed of a breathing bag, appropriate connecting pieces, and a nasal mask or cannula (Fig. 7-12) and is connected to a common outflow tube from the mixing chamber of the machine.

Breathing bag. The purpose of the breathing bag is to provide a reservoir for gases to be inhaled from the system. It should be large enough to accommodate a volume equivalent to the average adult lung capacity (4 to 6 liters). The total flow of gases through the flowmeter should be adjusted so as to keep

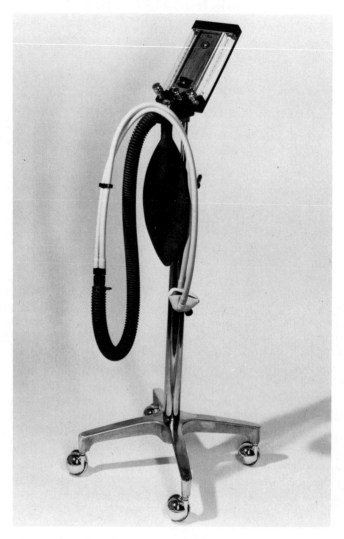

Fig. 7-12. Mobile analgesia machine with inhaler assembly attached. (Courtesy Fraser Sweatman, Inc.)

the breathing bag from collapsing even during the patient's greatest inspiratory effort.

Connecting pieces. A single rubber tubing is used to connect the breathing bag to the nasal mask or cannula. This tubing may be of varying lengths to accommodate the needs of the practitioner. Since all analgesia machines use a nonrebreathing system (see next section), there will not be an increase in dead space.

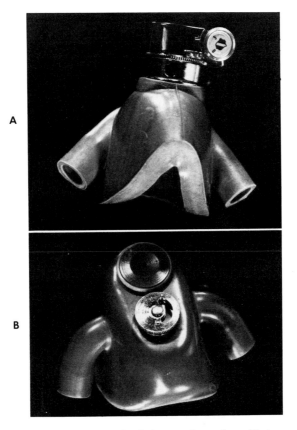

Fig. 7-13. Nasal mask. **A,** With metal exhalation valve and air dilution port. **B,** With lightweight rubber exhalation valve and metal air dilution port.

Nasal mask. The nasal mask (Fig. 7-13), frequently referred to as a nasal hood or nasal inhaler, is available in various sizes and is designed to fit the facial contour closely and to have a soft rim or cushion along the area of contact, both to make a tight, leakproof application and at the same time not injure the face.

The nasal mask is equipped with two valves that, depending on the manufacturer, may or may not be adjustable. These valves are an exhalation valve and an air dilution valve or port.

Exhalation valve. Whenever nitrous oxide–oxygen conscious-sedation is being employed, the exhalation valve must be adjusted to the *wide open* position at all times. It is through the use of this valve that the analgesia machine is considered to utilize a nonrebreathing system. That is, the flow of gases is from the machine to the patient and from the patient to the atmosphere. With the use of the nonrebreathing system, the cost and inconvenience of a circle system (see below), as well as the possibility of carbon dioxide accumulation to excess, are eliminated. The patient always breathes "fresh" gases as they are delivered from the machine.

Air dilution valve or port. The nasal mask is also equipped with an air dilution valve or port, which can be adjusted from a fully open to a fully closed position. Although differences of opinion exist concerning the position of this valve, it is my belief that the valve should remain closed at all times during the production of conscious-sedation. My reasons for this are quite simple. First, nitrous oxide is an extremely weak agent that diffuses quite rapidly. This means that an effective concentration will be difficult or impossible to attain if there are leaks between connections or between the mask and the patient's face.

The purpose of the air dilution valve is to allow the patient to breathe a mixture of nitrous oxide, oxygen, and room air. The presence of room air in the mixture supposedly ensures the safety of the system. However, a system that is operated with the air dilution valve open is also ineffective.

Second, with the air dilution valve wide open and the machine delivering 50% nitrous oxide and 50% oxygen, the patient has been shown to be inhaling between 15% and 17% nitrous oxide at the maximum. When the valve is partly open, the concentration of nitrous oxide in the inhaled mixture is unknown. It is my belief that when any drugs are administered one must be aware of the dose (concentration) that he is delivering. Only with the air dilution valve closed is this possible when one is administering nitrous oxide and oxygen.

Third, it is economically unwise to administer nitrous oxide and oxygen with the air dilution valve open. The difference between the 50% that the machine is delivering and the 15% that the patient is actually inhaling is merely diffusing into the room and being wasted. If the desired effect is obtainable with a concentration as low as 15%, it is my belief that the air dilution valve should be closed and the flowmeters adjusted to deliver 15% nitrous oxide and 85% oxygen. In this manner a known dose (concentration) is being delivered to the patient while economically producing the desired results.

Recently much concern has been shown over the possible harmful effects of trace contaminants within the dental operatory on office personnel. Included among these contaminants is nitrous oxide. Studies are being carried out to determine whether or not chronic exposure to trace amounts of this agent is capable of producing deleterious effects.

Although numerous animal studies and retrospective surveys involving humans have suggested a cause and effect relationship to date, no well-documented studies exist demonstrating any long-term ill effects in humans from chronic exposure to trace amounts of nitrous oxide.

It is thought by some that this trace contaminant presents a potential

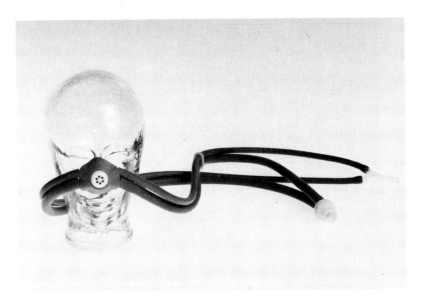

Fig. 7-14. Scavenging nasal mask. (Courtesy Narco McKesson.)

health hazard that should be regulated and controlled. The National Institute for Occupational Safety and Health states that with proper scavenging equipment, room levels of 30 parts per million nitrous oxide "can be obtained," yet it readily admits that this amount cannot be considered to be a "safe" level since the dangers of chronic exposure have not yet been defined.

Nevertheless, devices are appearing on the market to assure exposure of office personnel to lowest amounts possible. The most popular, inexpensive, and effective device is the scavenging nasal mask (Fig. 7-14). In contrast to the conventional mask/tubing arrangement, the mask is adapted with two inhalation tubes that exhaust the expired gas mixture from the operatory by way of a suction system. In this manner a nonrebreathing system is maintained yet trace amounts of nitrous oxide are less apt to accumulate in the atmosphere.

Nasal cannula. A nasal cannula (Fig. 7-15) rather than a nasal mask is available for the delivery of nitrous oxide and oxygen mixtures to be inhaled by the patient. The cannula is less cumbersome than the nasal mask and has been advocated by some for this reason.

The cannula is made of soft rubber or plastic and has projections that fit into each nostril. However, the cannula does not fit snugly into the nostril and allows the patient to inhale room air as well as nitrous oxide and oxygen. For this reason, sufficient concentrations of nitrous oxide may not be obtainable unless high flows of gases are delivered from the machine.

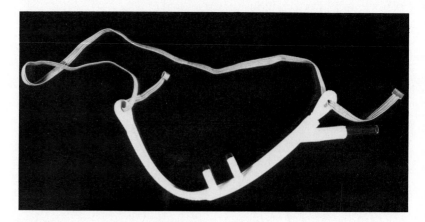

Fig. 7-15. Nasal cannula.

It has been demonstrated that with the use of the nasal cannula the administration of more than 25% nitrous oxide is not possible unless the machine delivers less than 20% oxygen, a feat not possible with modern analgesia machines.

The economic disadvantage of the nasal connula is self-evident. In addition, the high flows of dry gases into the nostrils and nasopharynx cause a degree of desiccation of the tissues that is uncomfortable if the procedure is of more than brief duration.

Nevertheless, the nasal cannula, being less cumbersome than a nasal mask, is a worthwhile and inexpensive piece of equipment that may prove to be invaluable on selected patients.

ANALGESIA MACHINE VERSUS ANESTHETIC MACHINE

Most machines marketed today for the production of conscious-sedation with the use of nitrous oxide are termed *analgesia* machines, to distinguish them from *anesthetic* machines, which are used for the production of general anesthesia. The machines resemble each other in many respects, yet certain important differences are present and must be discussed.

Minimum oxygen flow

Each analgesia machine is designed to deliver a certain minimum flow of oxygen. The minimum flow rate is preset by the manufacturer and is immediately established once the machine is turned on. For most models the minimum oxygen flow rate is betwen 3 and 5 liters per minute.

This is in contrast to an anesthesia machine, which has no "on-off" switch and in which the oxygen flow may be adjusted from 0 to over 12 liters per minute.

Once the analgesia machine is turned on and the minimum oxygen flow established, the valve controlling the flow of nitrous oxide will be effective in establishing the flow of this gas. Unless the machine is in the "on" position and the minimum oxygen flow established, nitrous oxide cannot be delivered.

Through the use of the minimum oxygen flow mechanism the practitioner is prevented from intentionally or inadvertently administering 100% nitrous oxide.

Fail safe system

Coupled with the minimum oxygen flow system is a "fail safe" system that automatically shuts off the nitrous oxide flow in the event that the oxygen flow rate should fall below the preset minimum for any reason (for example, depletion of this oxygen source resulting from consumption of the gas in a cylinder). Under these circumstances it would again be impossible for the practitioner to deliver 100% nitrous oxide to the patient. The available gas supply to the patient from the machine being dicontinued, normal physiological function would cause the patient to resume breathing room air through his mouth.

Maximum nitrous oxide concentration

Once again, because of the minimum oxygen flow rate that is established when an analgesia machine is turned on, the maximum nitrous oxide concentration deliverable is limited to around 80%. By virtue of the fact that a certain minimum flow of oxygen is established when the machine is turned on, delivering nitrous oxide at the maximum flow possible (usually about 10 liters per minute) limits its concentration to less than 80%, the remainder being oxygen.

Since room air contains about 20% oxygen, various manufacturers tout the safety of their device by claiming that one cannot deliver less than the amount of oxygen required for normal metabolic function. The implication of safety in this regard is highly overrated. Adequate oxygenation of tissues depends not only on an adequate oxygen concentration in the inspired air but also on the free movement of air into and out of the ventilating portion of the lungs. Most certainly, administration of 80% nitrous oxide and 20% oxygen will result in the production of unconsciousness. The likelihood of airway obstruction and partial or complete interference with ventilation is almost sure to materialize in the hands of one unfamiliar with management of the unconscious patient.

For this reason one must not allow his patient to lose consciousness for even a brief period of time, regardless of the oxygen concentration in the inspired mixture.

Management of office emergencies including the unconscious patient will be discussed in Chapter 11.

Nonrebreathing system

All analgesia machines currently available employ a nonrebreathing system (Magill circuit) for the delivery of gases to the patient. This is in contrast to anesthetic machines, in which a partial rebreathing system is usually employed.

The nonrebreathing system delivers gas from the machine via a single breathing tube to the patient. The patient's exhalations pass into the atmosphere through an exhalation valve.

In a system involving partial rebreathing, the patient's exhalations pass back into the breathing circle through a second breathing tube. Carbon dioxide is removed by a cannister containing a chemical compound to absorb this, and after oxygen is added the patient rebreathes the remaining portion of the previously exhaled gas mixture.

Thus the anesthetic machine possesses two breathing tubes, one for inhalation and the other for exhalation, and a carbon dioxide absorber.

Although a rebreathing system can be employed for the production of conscious-sedation, a nonrebreathing system is preferable. Equipment is less cumbersome, the need for cannister changes is eliminated, and carbon dioxide retention by the patient is not likely to occur. Since exhaled gases are eliminated from the system rather than being rebreathed, this system is somewhat more expensive to operate. However, the advantages to be gained more than offset any additional cost that may be incurred.

Flush valve

All the analgesia as well as the anesthetic machines currently marketed have a flush valve or knob that, when turned on, fills the breathing bag with 100% oxygen at a flow of about 50 liters per minute. This device enables one to rapidly fill the system with pure oxygen when desired. In this manner either machine may be used as a manual resuscitator if required.

CARE OF EQUIPMENT

Care should be taken to protect the analgesia machine from abuse that might alter its functional characteristics. Most machines are made of metal, plastic, and glass and are quite durable in ordinary usage. As with the cylinders, regulators, and valves, no oil or grease should come in contact with any part of the machine itself.

The rubber goods of the inhaler assembly require a minimum amount of care. Simple precautions can be taken to prolong their cleanliness and durability.

Rubber is damaged by exposure to light, particularly sunlight and ultraviolet light, by heat, and by contact with oils and greases. When stored, the articles should be kept in an unstrained condition. They should lie flat, without creases or bends.

On completion of every procedure the mask, bag, and tubing should be sanitized by washing with soap and water and then thoroughly rinsed at least three times. Most organisms can be effectively eliminated by these methods. No injury to the equipment or the patient has been encountered.

One should remember to apply the common principles of cleanliness in caring for those items of the analgesia equipment through which a patient's breath will pass and which will come in contact with the patient.

At the end of each day those machines using a portable gas source or a regulator system in which flexible tubing is connected directly to the analgesia unit should have both gases turned off at their source while the machine and its flowmeters are turned on. This maneuver "bleeds" the line pressure to zero and eliminates all gas that might otherwise contribute to a fire of unrelated origin. Disconnecting a machine from the wall outlet accomplishes the same end when a manifold system is utilized.

Chapter 8

THE PHARMACOLOGY OF
CONSCIOUS-SEDATIVE AGENTS

Although numerous agents may be used, either alone or in combination, and may be administered by several routes for the production of conscious-sedation, for the purpose of discussion they may be placed into four categories as follows:

1. Psychosedatives
2. Barbiturate and nonbarbiturate sedatives
3. Narcotic analgetics
4. Belladonna derivatives

Drugs in each category have specific qualities that make them useful in the production of conscious-sedation. Some have limitations and disadvantages, which must also be understood if one is to be able to derive full benefit from conscious-sedative techniques.

Only through a thorough understanding of the pharmacology of drugs in each category is the dentist able to select the agent or agents that can provide conscious-sedation with one of its chief attributes, versatility.

PSYCHOSEDATIVES

Psychosedative agents are those drugs that heretofore have been referred to as tranquilizers. Dentists should refrain from the use of this term, since it is a layman's name for an agent that does not exist; the true "tranquilizer" has not yet been developed.

Chemistry. Those agents classified as psychosedatives may be further subdivided into major and minor psychosedative drugs.

Major psychosedatives are those agents that are useful in the treatment and management of psychotic patients. Most agents of usefulness in this category are phenothiazine derivatives, the most popular being propiomazine (Largon) and promethazine (Phenergan) (Fig. 8-1).

Minor psychosedatives are those nonphenothiazine agents that are useful

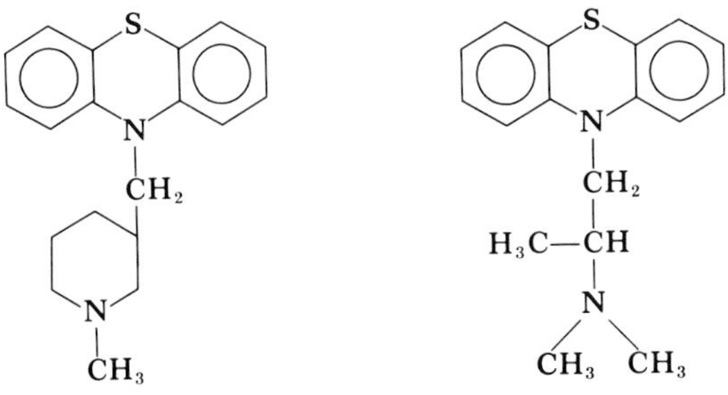

Fig. 8-1. A, Propiomazine (Largon). **B,** Promethazine (Phenergan).

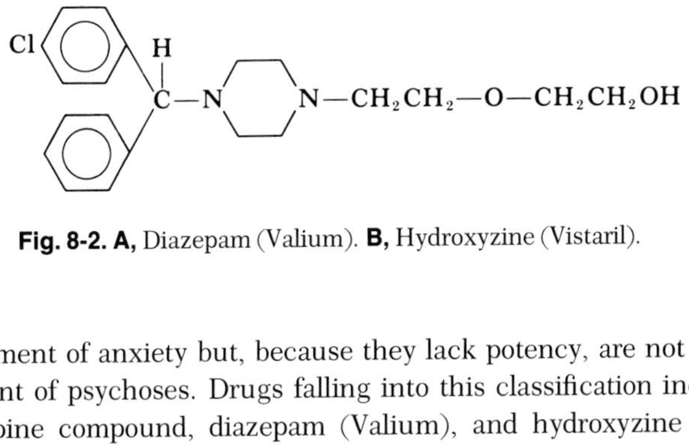

Fig. 8-2. A, Diazepam (Valium). **B,** Hydroxyzine (Vistaril).

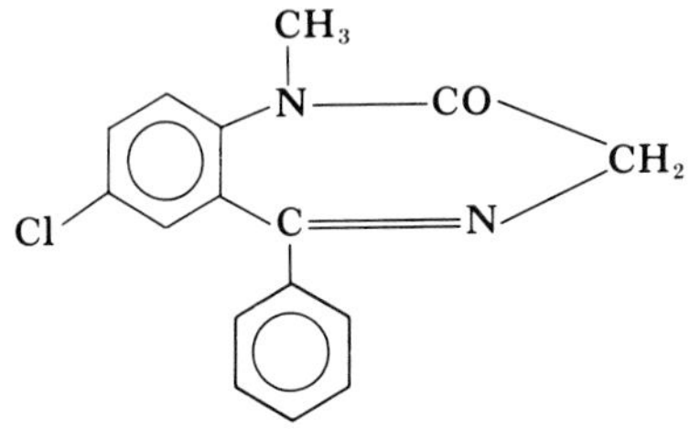

in the treatment of anxiety but, because they lack potency, are not useful in the treatment of psychoses. Drugs falling into this classification include the benzodiazepine compound, diazepam (Valium), and hydroxyzine (Vistaril) (Fig. 8-2).

Pharmacology. Whether the agent is a major or a minor psychosedative, the pharmacological effects are similar, varying mainly in intensity. Although these agents have been demonstrated to possess a wide variety of properties, including antihistaminic, antiemetic, and local anesthetic actions, their main pharmacological effect is on all levels of the cerebrospinal axis. Apparently their greatest effect, that of calming and sedating, occurs through an action on the reticular activating system of the brainstem and other subcortical centers. In contrast to barbiturates, they exert very little effect on the cerebral cortex.

Through their effect on these centers the drugs are able to modify behavior by producing psychomotor slowing, emotional quieting, and indifference to environmental stimuli while producing little ataxia, incoordination, or alteration of cognitive ability. Even for these reasons alone, the psychosedative agents would be useful in the production of conscious-sedation. However, their greatest benefit lies in their ability to potentiate the action of barbiturates and narcotic analgetics. When those agents are used in conjunction with psychosedative drugs, their full effects may be achieved with lower dosages than would be required in the absence of the psychosedative agents.

The psychosedative drugs also have effects on the cardiovascular system that must be considered. Through their direct actions on the heart and blood vessels and actions on the central nervous system and autonomic reflexes one may produce hypotensive effects, particularly with the use of the major psychosedatives. This is especially true if the drugs are administered rapidly via the intravenous route. This complication will not be seen if the drugs are administered slowly and in small increments rather than in a bolus.

Regardless of the rate and the route of administration, however, postural hypotension, or hypotension produced by changing to the erect position, is a distinct possibility in patients who have received psychosedative drugs. For this reason all patients should be instructed to sit erect and then to stand erect slowly at the end of the appointment.

Clinical considerations. The psychosedative agents are useful adjuncts for the control of fear and apprehension in many patients. The patients who are only mildly or moderately apprehensive may be managed with the use of a psychosedative alone. Patients exhibiting a greater degree of anxiety may be managed with a combination of a psychosedative plus a narcotic analgetic and/or a barbiturate.

Practically all psychosedatives can be given orally, subcutaneously, intramuscularly, or intravenously. For most efficient usage the intravenous route is the method of choice. Because of these agents' potential effects on the cardiovascular system small incremental doses should be administered while observing (titrating) the patient to produce the desired effect.

Aid should be provided to the patient in standing at the end of the appointment. He must not be permitted to stand quickly and walk from the operatory unassisted; postural hypotension, dizziness, weakness, and stumbling or falling might occur. Patients should be cautioned to sit or stand up slowly and deliberately for several hours after the appointment. In my experience, postural changes following the conservative doses of drugs for conscious-sedation have not caused these symptoms to appear.

The agents that I have found to be most useful in the production of conscious-sedation include promethazine (Phenergan), propiomazine (Largon), and diazepam (Valium) in intravenous doses of 25 to 50 mg., 10 to 20 mg., and 2.5 to 20 mg., respectively.

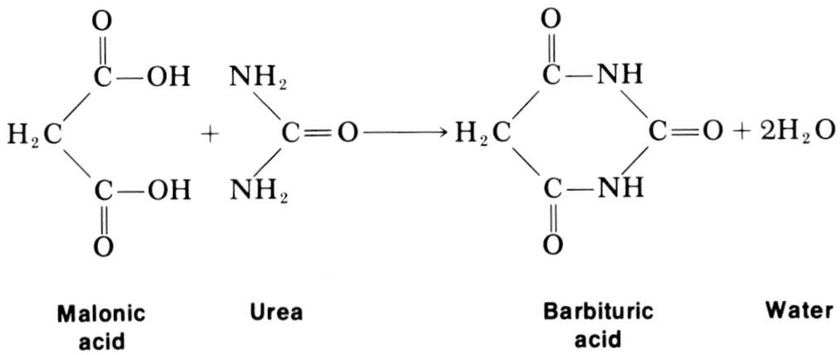

Fig. 8-3. Barbituric acid (malonic acid–urea).

Although hydroxyzine (Vistaril) is useful intramuscularly in doses up to 100 mg., it is not recommended for intravenous use at this time.

BARBITURATE AND NONBARBITURATE SEDATIVES
Barbiturates

Chemistry. Barbiturates are those agents that may pharmacologically be described as "sedative-hypnotics." Chemically, they are derivatives of barbituric acid or malonyl urea, which is a combination of malonic acid and urea (Fig. 8-3).

Barbituric acid itself has no hypnotic properties, but replacement of hydrogen by various radicals produces many different drugs possessing hypnotic characteristics. The new compounds are varied in their actions, both the potency and duration of action being markedly affected by the different substitutions. According to Goodman and Gilman over 2,500 barbiturates have been prepared.

Pharmacology. The barbiturates may be divided into two categories on the basis of chemical structure. Those compounds having an oxygen attached to the carbon of the urea component are properly termed *barbiturates*. They are frequently referred to as oxybarbiturates to distinguish them from those of the second category, the thiobarbiturates—which have a sulfur atom in place of the oxygen. Although the pharmacology of all barbiturates is essentially similar they differ in potency, duration, and intensity of effect. Thiobarbiturates possess a greater degree of fat solubility, are more rapid in onset, have a shorter duration of action, and are somewhat more toxic than the oxybarbiturates.

The barbiturates are general depressants; they depress the activity of nerve, skeletal muscle, smooth muscle, cardiac muscle, and the central nervous system. However, it must be emphasized that the central nervous system is exquisitely sensitive to depression by barbiturates; as a result, when these drugs are administered in therapeutic doses, the effects on other structures are absent or negligible. All degrees of depression of the central nervous system are possible, ranging from mild sedation to general anesthesia or to coma and death.

The primary site of action of the barbiturates is not completely understood. Attempts have been made to localize the action of these agents to certain gross areas of the brainstem such as the midbrain tegmentum or hypothalamus. Drugs in this category appear to act at all levels of the neuraxis. Nevertheless, there is a complex, interrelated group of pathways coursing through the reticular formation of the midbrain and medulla and extending anteriorly into the thalamus and hypothalamus—the "reticular activating system." This system is very sensitive to the depressant effects of sedative-hypnotic drugs. It is their effect on the reticular system that seems to be responsible for the inability to maintain wakefulness under the influence of these compounds. It would also seem logical to assume that the cerebral cortex is among structures most sensitive to these drugs, since they do depress cerebral function—as evidenced by release of inhibitions and the production of amnesia in the conscious patient.

In doses that would ordinarily be used for conscious-sedation, the barbiturates have an extremely low incidence of untoward reactions, with no significant depressant effect on respiration or circulation. Larger doses usually depress respirations and may cause a sharp fall in blood pressure. In therapeutic doses the barbiturates do not affect the heart muscle or cardiac output.

The drugs lack the ability to obtund the sense of pain without definite impairment of consciousness. They cannot be classified as analgetic agents and when given alone have been shown to lower the pain threshold rather than elevate it. They cannot be relied on to relieve pain of any degree in the conscious patient, not will they produce sedation in the presence of even mild pain. For this reason one must never rely on barbiturates to compensate for poor regional analgesia or to eliminate the need for control of pain perception. This can be accomplished only by rendering the patient unconscious.

Untoward reactions to small doses of barbiturates are extremely rare. Toxic symptoms may be encountered in a particularly sensitive patient who becomes unduly affected by a small dose of the drug. Symptoms will be manifested by a greater degree of sedation than desired and, possibly, sleep. Respiratory depression will result only from an overdose and is in direct proportion to the amount administered. This should never be allowed to occur in a patient under conscious-sedation, since all medications will be administered in very small aliquots qhile the patient is being observed for drug effects.

Termination of activity. Three processes are responsible for terminating the central nervous system effects of the barbiturates: physical redistribution, metabolic degradiation, and renal excretion. All three mechanisms cause a decrease in the plasma level and result in withdrawal of the agent from the central nervous system.

Long-acting agents such as phenobarbital are excreted unchanged by the kidney. Short-acting agents such as pentobarbital (Nembutal) undergo biotransformation by the liver and excretion of resultant products by the kidney.

Except for those long-acting agents excreted unchanged by the kidney, all barbiturates undergo rather slow biotransformation, about 20% per hour.

The role of redistribution in termination of activity is most important when one considers the ultrashort-acting barbiturates, which are highly fat-soluble. Rapid emergence from effects with these agents is due to their physical redistribution to nonsensitive fatty tissue.

Because of a high perfusion rate the brain, which receives about 30% of the cardiac output, also receives a maximum concentration of intravenously administered barbiturate in about 30 seconds. Following this initial and rapid effect, the drug equilibrates over the next few minutes with other fatty, less well perfused tissues. Hence, central nervous system levels fall and effects terminate. A further decline in plasma concentration occurs as a result of biotransformation and excretion.

It is imperative, therefore, that patients who have received barbiturates be escorted from the office by a responsible adult. Even though the drug effect may appear to be terminated, residual amounts will usually be present in sufficient quantity to impair sensory perception to a mild degree.

The patient with an impaired cardiovascular, respiratory, or hepatic system should be given a proportionately smaller dose of barbiturates. It is extremely doubtful that any ambulatory patient able to present himself in the dental office would have a sufficiently impaired hepatic or renal system to be unable to degrade and eliminate these drugs.

In addition, while not specifically contraindicated, barbiturates should be administered in small increments and with careful observation of those patients having severely compromised cardiovascular and respiratory systems.

About the only valid contraindications to the use of barbiturates would be a history of allergy to them or the presence of porphyria.

Types. It has been mentioned that the various barbiturates are similar in effects and differ mainly in their time of onset and duration of action. On this basis they are divided into four groups:

1. Ultrashort-acting
2. Short-acting
3. Intermediate-acting
4. Long-acting

Ultrashort-acting barbiturates. The ultrashort-acting barbiturates most commonly used are thiopental sodium (Pentothal), thiamylal sodium (Surital), and methohexital sodium (Brevital). With the exception of thiopental these drugs are administered exclusively by the intravenous route for the production of conscious-sedation. And though they possess the shortest duration of action, they are also the most potent barbiturates available. Unconsciousness and general anesthesia may be produced with as little as 50 mg. of methohexital administered intravenously to an otherwise unmedicated patient. Smaller doses may have similar effects in patients already under the influence of other central nervous system—depressing drugs.

It is for this reason that only extremely small doses (in the range of 5 mg.)

should be administered, with the patient being observed for pharmacological effects. An adequate amount of time for peak drug effect must be allowed to elapse before subsequent doses follow. With all drugs in this group the peak effect after intravenous administration will be realized in 30 to 60 seconds. Sedative effects will be present for 5 to 7 minutes for methohexital, the shortest-acting and most potent barbiturate, and for 10 to 15 minutes with thiopental and thiamylal.

Thiopental is the only agent in this group that may be administered by any route other than the intravenous. A rectal suspension is available that when instilled rectally in doses of no more than 10 to 14 mg. per pound will produce sedation in 8 to 10 minutes. This method is particularly useful in apprehensive children. Duration will be about 30 to 60 minutes.

Ultrashort-acting barbiturates are particularly useful when performing dental procedures which are of very brief duration. They are also quite useful for providing amnesia of short duration. For example, a state of conscious-sedation may be produced by using psychosedative and/or a narcotic analgetic. With the patient in a calmed and relaxed state, small increments of methohexital may be administered to produce amnesia for the application of regional analgesia, a tooth extraction, or any other particularly annoying procedure that is not time-consuming. It must be stressed, however, that operative pain control is *always* provided by *adequate regional analgesia*.

Short-acting barbiturates. The short-acting barbiturates most commonly used are pentobarbital (Nembutal) and secobarbital (Seconal). They may be administered orally, intramuscularly, or intravenously.

These drugs are particularly useful via the intravenous route for the production of conscious-sedation, either as the sole agent or in combination with other central nervous system depressants. When used alone the intravenous dose range will usually be from 50 to 100 mg. Lower doses must be employed when used these drugs are used in conjunction with psychosedatives and/or narcotic analgetics. Duration of sedation via the intravenous route will range from 2 to 3 hours while amnesic effects may persist for 30 to 45 minutes.

Short-acting barbiturates are also of value when administered via the oral route to provide the patient with a restful sleep the night before his dental appointment. Depending on the individual, the oral dose will range from 50 to 200 mg. The drug will require 30 to 45 minutes for its maximum effectiveness and will have a duration of 4 to 6 hours. Providing the patient with a restful sleep the night before his appointment will allow him to arrive at the office well rested and thus with an elevated pain reaction threshold.

Intermediate-acting barbiturates. The intermediate-acting barbiturates most commonly used are amobarbital (Amytal), aprobarbital (Alurate), and butabarbital (Butisol). They are administered via the oral route only and effective in 45 minutes to 1 hour. Duration will range from 6 to 8 hours. They may be

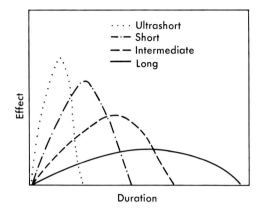

Fig. 8-4. Relationship between duration and intensity of effect, for categories of barbiturates.

used to best advantage on the night before the appointment to aid the patient in obtaining a good night's rest. The dose will differ with the individual patient, varying from 50 to 100 mg.

Long-acting barbiturates. The long-acting barbiturates most commonly used are barbital sodium and phenobarbital (Luminal). These agents are indicated for oral administration only and, because of their long duration of 8 to 10 hours, are seldom if ever indicated in dental practice.

Duration. As pointed out, the duration of barbiturates varies widely. "Duration" does not imply that peak effectiveness of the drug is maintained for that entire period of time; however, the drug may produce enough effect over a period of time to interfere with normal judgment and coordination. This must be considered when prescribing or administering the various barbiturates and instructing the patients as to their activities while under the influence of these drugs.

Another fact to be considered is that, when administered in therapeutic doses, the very short-acting barbiturates have very pronounced effect, whereas the long-acting agents have rather mild effects (Fig. 8-4).

Nonbarbiturate hypnotics

Although many nonbarbiturate hypnotics are currently available, they differ very little from barbiturates in pharmacological effects. They are of little value in conscious-sedation except in those cases in which the oral route of administration is preferred or an allergy to barbiturates necessitates their use. Their primary value lies in their ability to produce a restful night's sleep prior to the dental appointment. Peak effect occurs in about 30 to 45 minutes with a duration of 4 to 6 hours.

Popular nonbarbiturates and their oral dosages are the following:

Chloral hydrate (Noctec)	500 to 1,000 mg.
Ethchlorvynol (Placidyl)	500 to 750 mg.
Glutethimide (Doriden)	240 to 500 mg.
Methaqualone (Quaalude)	150 to 300 mg.

NARCOTIC ANALGETICS

Narcotic analgetics are particularly useful drugs in the production of conscious-sedation. In addition to their excellent ability to elevate the pain threshold, through actions on central nervous system centers, they also have a definite, though mild, depressing effect on the cerebral cortex. Not only are they useful in elevating the pain threshold but they are also capable of significantly altering the patient's mood, providing freedom from fear of pain as well.

Many narcotic analgetics are available for use in conscious-sedation techniques. Their pharmacological effects are quite similar. However, wide variances are seen in their duration and potency. Both naturally occurring and synthetic agents that are available and quite useful in dental practice will be discussed; the names of other, less useful agents will be included for completeness only.

The narcotic analgetics may be divided into three groups: (1) opiates or alkaloids of opium, which include morphine, Pantopon, and codeine; (2) the synthetic opiates, which include dihydromorphinone (Dilaudid), diacetylmorphine (heroin), dihydrohydroxymorphinone (Numorphan), and methyldihydromorphinone (Metopon); and (3) opioids, or synthetic compounds, which include meperidine (Demerol), alphaprodine (Nisentil), methadone (Dolophine), levo-dromoran (Levorphan), anileridine (Leritine), and fentanyl (Sublimaze).

Opiates or alkaloids of opium

The naturally occurring narcotic analgetics are obtained from opium, which is in turn obtained from the milky exudate of the Oriental poppy seed. This exudate contains many alkaloids, of which 75% are resins and oils pharmacologically unfit for use. About 10% of opium is morphine, whereas codeine represents about 0.5%.

Morphine

Morphine is the standard of comparison for all narcotic analgetics and typifies the pharmacology for this group of drugs. For this reason it will be discussed in greater detail than the others.

Chemistry. Morphine is the principal alkaloid of opium and has the following formula: $C_{17}H_{19}NO_3 + H_2O$ (Fig. 8-5).

Pharmacology. The most outstanding characteristic of morphine is the

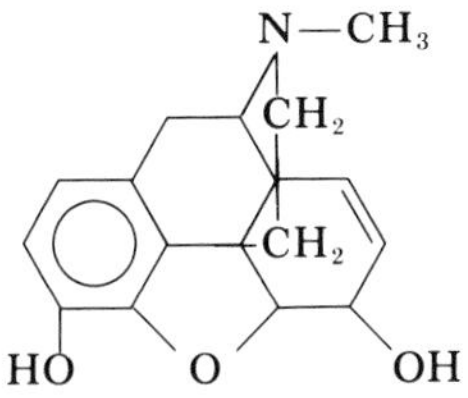

Fig. 8-5. Morphine.

production of analgesia. And, although the exact central nervous system site of action is unknown, morphine is believed to have a selective action on the pain centers in the optic thalami. The analgetic effect results strictly from actions on the central nervous system, thus altering pain reaction. The opioids neither alter the threshold or responsiveness of nerve endings to noxious stimulation nor impair the conduction of the nerve impulse along peripheral nerves.

Analgesia is accompanied by drowsiness, changes in mood, and mental clouding. The extremities feel heavy and the body warm, the face (and especially the nose) may itch, and the mouth becomes dry. In doses of 3 to 15 mg. morphine rarely produces amnesia but most frequently produces euphoria and an unrealistic sense of well-being. Mental clouding is characterized by an inability to concentrate, difficulty in mentation, apathy, lessened physical activity, reduced visual acuity, and lethargy.

On occasion the administration of morphine does not result in a pleasant experience. Sometimes dysphoria, consisting of mild anxiety, agitation, fear, and occasionally nausea and vomiting, rather than euphoria results. Dysphoria can usually be controlled by the use of a psychosedative agent. Although mention of dysphoria was thought to be an important consideration, its clinical occurrence in the production of conscious-sedation is insignificant.

The pupils usually constrict in the patients who have received a single dose of morphine. In morphine poisoning, the miosis is marked and pinpoint pupils are pathognomonic. Tolerance to this effect does not occur, and the morphine addict continues to have constricted pupils.

Respiration will be depressed in direct proportion to the dose and the susceptibility of the patient, with maximum depression occurring approximately 7 minutes after intravenous administration. The mechanism of respiratory depression by narcotic analgetics is through a reduction in the responsiveness of the respiratory center to increases in carbon dioxide concentration. Death resulting from overdose is usually due to respiratory depression and resultant asphyxia. All narcotic analgetics should be used with care in any patients in whom even mild respiratory depression might not be well tolerated. Among those are included patients with emphysema, kyphoscoliosis, and obesity.

Morphine and related drugs have little or no effect on the cardiovascular system. Changes that do occur in blood pressure or pulse rate are secondary to psychological effects and lessened physical activity. The vasomotor center is not affected even by those doses that cause obvious respiratory depression.

It should be noted, however, that morphine and most other narcotic analgetics decrease the capacity of the cardiovascular system to respond to the stress of gravitational shifts. Thus when the supine patient stands erect, orthostatic hypotension due to peripheral vasodilation may occur.

All narcotics have the limited ability to produce nausea and vomiting by stimulation of the chemoreceptor trigger zone in the medulla. Phenothiazine psychosedative agents have the ability to block this effect.

Goodman and Gilman state that nausea occurs in approximately 40% and vomiting in 16% of ambulatory patients receiving morphine. This has not been my experience. I have yet to see a properly prepared ambulatory patient vomit and have seen nausea on very few occasions after the intravenous administration of any narcotic analgetic.

The major pathway for the biotransformation of morphine is conjugation with glucuronic acid by the liver and excretion by the kidneys as monoglucuronide.

Morphine may be administered intravenously, intramuscularly, or subcutaneously in doses ranging from 3 to 15 mg. The drug is not active when administered by the oral route. A duration of about 2 hours may be expected after intravenous administration.

Synthetic opiates

The synthetic opiates include agents that are either illegal or not practical for conscious-sedation because of their prolonged action. Among these are diacetylmorphine (heroin), dihydromorphinone, dihydrohydroxymorphine, and methyldihydromorphinone.

Opioids or synthetic compounds

The opioids, or synthetic compounds, are among the most popular agents for the production of conscious-sedation. They may be employed alone or in combination with other agents and may be administered by several routes.

Meperidine (Demerol)

Meperidine is ethyl 1-methyl-4-phenylpiperidine-4-carboxylate hydrochloride (Fig. 8-6) and is the first synthetic narcotic analgetic and opioid. It is a white, odorless crystal that is soluble in water and has a slightly bitter taste. It can be administered orally, intramuscularly, or intravenously in 50 to 100 mg. doses, but it is not recommended for subcutaneous use.

Meperidine possesses the combined properties of morphine and atropine and has an analgetic potency somewhat less than that of morphine. In average doses it is capable of raising the pain threshold by 60% to 65%.

In equianalgetic doses, meperidine produces as much sedation, euphoria,

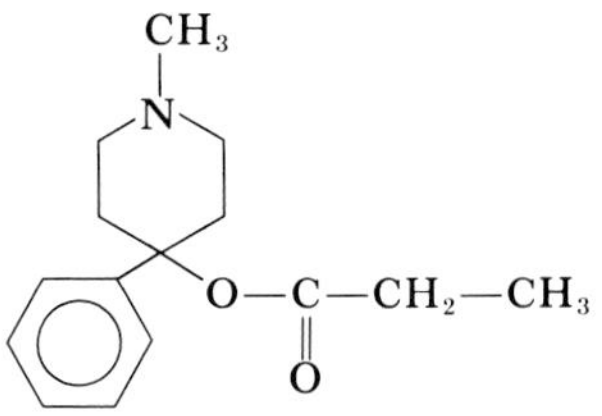

Fig. 8-6. Meperidine (Demerol).

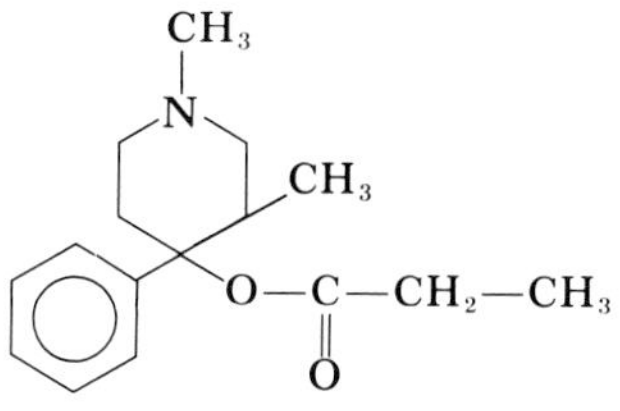

Fig. 8-7. Alphaprodine (Nisentil).

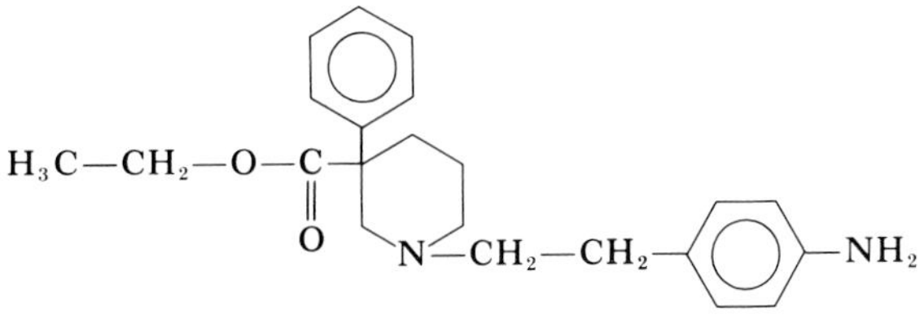

Fig. 8-8. Anileridine (Leritine).

mood alteration, and respiratory depression as morphine. Its duration of action is also comparable to that of morphine. But, unlike morphine, pupillary size and pupillary reflexes are not usually affected.

The drug produces little if any effect on the cardiovascular system, although postural hypotension may occur if an erect posture is assumed rapidly.

Dizziness is the most common complication in ambulatory patients. The drug undergoes biotransformation in the liver and excretion by the kidneys.

Alphaprodine (Nisentil)

Chemically, alphaprodine (Fig. 8-7) is dl-alpha-1,3-dimethyl-4-phenyl-4-proprionoxy-piperidine hydrochloride. It is a potent, short-acting narcotic analgetic capable of raising the pain threshold by 75% to 100%. The drug can be used both orally and parenterally and has a much more rapid onset than morphine or meperidine. The average adult dose is 40 to 60 mg.

Pharmacologically, alphaprodine is similar to meperidine in all respects. The advantages of this agent are its rapid onset, its short duration (about 45 minutes), its potency, and the fact that it is effective by any route of administration. The drug will usually be effective within 5 minutes regardless of its parenteral route of administration.

Anileridine (Leritine)

Anileridine is 1-(4-aminophenethyl)-4-phenylisonipectoic acid ethyl ester (Fig. 8-8). It is approximately two and one-half times as potent as meperidine and similar to it in its pharmacological effects and duration.

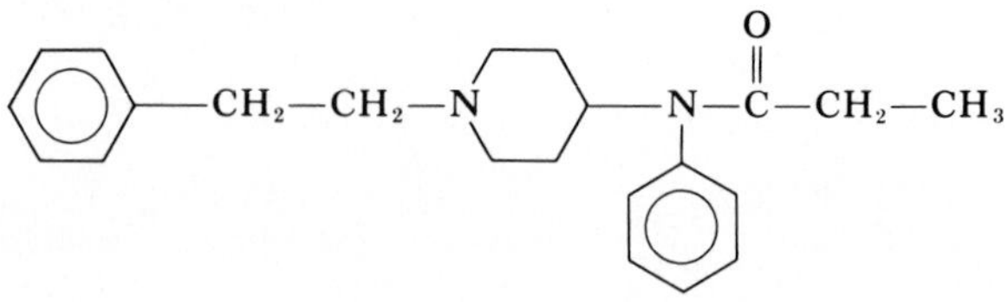

Fig. 8-9. Fentanyl (Sublimaze).

Fentanyl (Sublimaze)

Fentanyl, the newest and most potent narcotic analgetic to be introduced into clinical practice, is N-(1-phenethyl-4-piperidyl) propionanilide (Fig. 8-9). It is a derivative of meperidine and is 150 times as potent as morphine, which it resembles pharmacologically. Onset after intravenous administration is almost immediate, with maximal analgetic effect occurring within 3 to 5 minutes. Duration of action is about 30 minutes, making it the shortest-acting narcotic analgetic available. For this reason it is particularly well suited to use in ambulatory patients.

Dosages for use in ambulatory patients should be confined to 0.20 mg. (4 ml.) or less, given in 0.5 ml. increments. Higher doses or rapid administration of small doses may result in respiratory depression or apnea.

My experience with fentanyl has been rather extensive. On no occasion has respiratory depression been encountered using the conservative doses suggested.

Clinical considerations

Among those agents that may be used in the production of conscious-sedation, the narcotic analgetics are as near to ideal as any agent currently available. Their ability to alter the patient's mood and allay fear and apprehension is unparalleled.

When narcotic analgetics are administered intravenously in small incremental doses during observation of the patient, almost all objectives of conscious-sedation may be met rapidly. The doses used for conscious-sedation are capable of providing a degree of analgesia in addition to producing a calmed, somewhat euphoric patient. Respiratory and cardiovascular system depression and the production of dysphoria or nausea and vomiting are practically nonexistent.

The narcotic analgetics may be used in conjunction with psycho-sedatives, sedative-hypnotics, and belladonna derivatives for a greater range of effects. Care should be exercised when narcotic analgetics and barbiturates are being used concomitantly. Mixtures of these drugs, either in the same syringe or in an intravenous administration set, results in the formation of a precipitate that should not be injected.

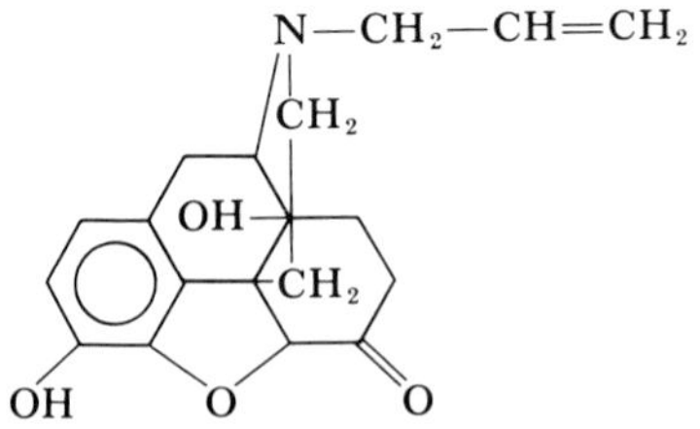

$$N-CH_2-CH=CH_2$$

Fig. 8-10. Naloxone (Narcan).

All persons using narcotic analgetics or certain other drugs that have an effect on the central nervous system must be aware of and comply with all regulations of the Controlled Substances Act of 1970.

NARCOTIC ANTAGONISTS

Every person using narcotic analgetics should be familar with the narcotic antagonists naloxone (Narcan) (Fig. 8-10), nalorphine (Nalline), and levallorphan (Lorfan). These have proved exceptionally useful in combating respiratory depression and other undesirable side effects of the narcotics. They are of no value as an antidote to the sedative-hypnotics but are dramatic in reversing the depressing effects of the narcotic analgetics.

Chemistry. The substitution of an allyl group for the N-methyl group in most narcotic analgetics such as morphine, levorphanol, and oxymorphone produces drugs with varying degrees of narcotic antagonistic effect. Thus nalorphine is a derivative of morphine whereas levallorphan and naloxone have levorphanol and oxymorphone, respectively, as their parent compounds.

Pharmacology. With the exception of naloxone the available narcotic antagonists have both antagonistic effects and varying degrees of agonistic activity. The effects of those agents with agonistic activity will depend on whether a narcotic has been previously administered. Agents that are partial agonists have the ability to produce autonomic and endocrine effects, analgesia, and respiratory depression in the absence of a narcotic analgetic. Naloxone, the one agent devoid of agonistic properties, produces no observable effect in the absence of a narcotic analgetic.

The most striking property of the narcotic antagonists is their marked ability to prevent or abolish many of the actions of narcotic analgetics. Narcotic-induced euphoria, dysphoria, analgesia, drowsiness, respiratory depression, muscular incoordination, vomiting, and miosis are all antagonized. This effect will be realized within 1 to 2 minutes after intravenous administration. The effect is believed to be achieved at a cellular level by competition for the same receptor site by the narcotic and its antagonist.

Levallorphan (5 mg.), nalorphine (1 mg.), or naloxone (0.4 mg.) given intravenously will effectively antagonize the therapeutic dose of any narcotic analgetic.

Clinical considerations. The narcotic antagonists are useful agents to have on hand whenever narcotic analgetics are being employed. However, judicious and proper use of narcotic analgetics should almost eliminate their need entirely except in the very rare individual who is particularly sensitive to the depressing effects of narcotic analgetics.

In the event that respiratory depression does occur, the narcotic antagonists must not be relied upon to ensure adequate ventilation. Theirs should be a secondary role. Ventilation must first be supported mechanically as described in Chapter 11. Nevertheless, their usefulness must not be understated in the management of respiratory depression.

As stated previously the narcotic antagonists are capable of antagonizing many narcotic analgetic effects, including drowsiness, analgesia, and respiratory depression. This does not mean that they are capable of completely reversing all effects to the extent that a patient previously administered a narcotic analgetic may be discharged from the office unescorted.

Some individuals advocate the combination of the narcotic analgetic with its antagonist for the production of conscious-sedation. Rationale for this combination is based on the premise that respiratory-depressing effects of the narcotic analgetic would be eliminated while desirable qualities would be allowed to remain. Personally, I do not favor this mixture for two reasons.

First, there will not be a significant amount of respiratory depression when narcotic analgetics are used for the production of conscious-sedation if both dose and rate of administration are properly controlled.

Second, narcotic antagonists have never been shown to be specific antagonists for the respiratory-depressing effects of the narcotic analgetics. All effects, including analgesia, euphoria, and the general sense of well-being, are antagonized by these agents. It would seem self-defeating, therefore, to administer one agent to produce a given set of pharmacological effects while simultaneously administering another agent to antagonize them.

BELLADONNA DERIVATIVES

The two naturally occuring belladonna derivatives that are of interest to the dentist are atropine and scopolamine. Due to similarities in pharmacology they will be discussed together, with pertinent differences noted.

Atropine and scopolamine

Chemistry. Atropine and scopolamine are organic bases that readily combine with acids to form salts. The salts are white crystalline powders, which are soluble in water and bitter to the taste. (See Figs. 8-11 and 8-12.)

Pharmacology. The belladonna alkaloids are useful in dentistry primarily for their ability to reduce the flow of saliva and thereby provide the dentist with

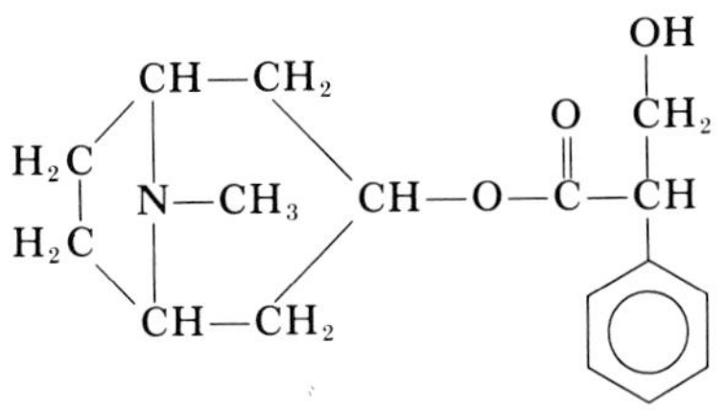

Fig. 8-11. Atropine.

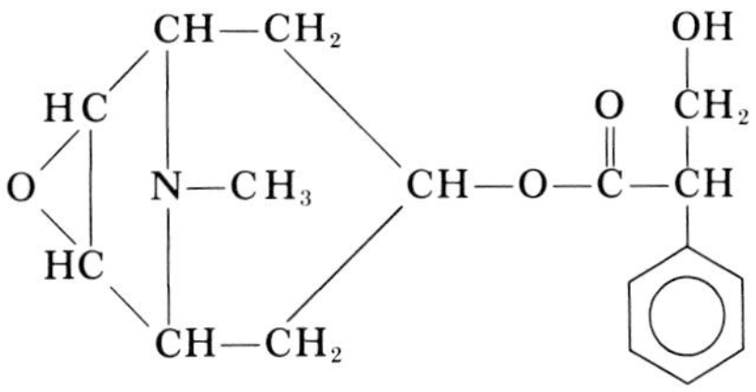

Fig. 8-12. Scopolamine.

a dry field in which to operate. Although these agents have many other actions, in my opinion their ability to reduce the flow of saliva should be their only use in conscious-sedative techniques.

In clinical doses atropine stimulates autonomic nerve fibers centrally and depresses them peripherally. In small doses it stimulates the medulla, particularly the vagus center, which produces bradycardia. Small doses also stimulate the respiratory center but have no effect on the cerebral cortex.

Atropine is used mainly for its peripheral effect in inhibiting the normal reactions produced by parasympathetic stimulation, which it annuls by competing with acetylcholine for receptor sites at the terminal ends of parasympathetic postganglionic nerver fibers.

Both atropine and scopolamine have the ability to increase heart rate and decrease salivary flow, with atropine being more potent in its effect on heart rate and scopolamine more potent as an antisialagogue.

The agents have approximately equal ability to paralyze the sphincter oculi muscle of the iris, causing dilation of the pupil. They also paralyze the ciliary muscle of the crystalline lens, causing photophobia and blurred vision for near objects.

On occasion atropine may cause a rash-like appearance on the skin of the neck and upper thorax. This anomalous vascular response results from dilation of cutaneous blood vessels of the blush area (atropine flush). It is frequently mistaken for allergic response to various medications.

Scopolamine, in contrast to atropine, is a central nervous depressant not unlike alcohol. The depression normally results in drowsiness, euphoria, amnesia, fatigue, and dreamless sleep. For these reasons it has been recommended as an adjunct to conscious-sedation.

However, the same doses occasionally cause excitement, restlessness, hallucinations, delirium, belligerent behavior, and prolonged amnesia. For these reasons I do not favor the use of scopolamine in the office patient undergoing conscious-sedation.

Clinical considerations. The primary role of the belladonna alkaloids in general dental practice is to decrease the flow of saliva, thus providing the dentist with a dry field in which to operate. Although the drug possess other qualities, which may be beneficial when general anesthesia is employed, those are not valid when conscious-sedation is being employed. While the drying effect of scopolamine is greater than that of atropine, it is of shorter duration.

Although the central nervous system–depressing effects of scopolamine are of great advantage in the majority of cases, the occasional production of excitement, hallucinations, and prolonged amnesia re sufficiently troublesome to contraindicate its use in the dental office.

Atropine and scopolamine may be administered by any route and will be effective within 5 minutes. A duration of about 1 to $1^{1}/_{2}$ hours may be expected.

NITROUS OXIDE

The chemistry, pharmacology, and clinical application of nitrous oxide are discussed in Chapter 6.

SUMMARY

Although no single agent exists that is capable of fulfilling all objectives of conscious-sedation, many drugs in several categories are available to meet selected requirements. through a knowledge of their attributes and shortcomings the dentist is able to select an infinite number of drug combinations and doses to design the conscious-sedative technique that is "just right" for each patient.

Through an understanding of the parmacology of *types* of drugs rather than specific agents the practitioner is better able to select those agents that fill the needs of patient and dentist alike. Thus safety and versatility in conscious-sedation are assured.

Chapter 9

TECHNICAL CONSIDERATIONS AND ROUTES OF ADMINISTRATION

If the use of conscious-sedation as a means of pain and apprehension control is to become an integral part of all phases of dental practice, one must not limit himself to the use of specific drugs or routes of administration. Rather, the dentist must familiarize himself with the "spectrum of pain control" as it pertains to conscious techniques and be able to select and combine the proper agents required to produce the desired result. Likewise, many avenues of drug administration are available. The dentist must be thoroughly familiar with their application in order to further enhance the versatility of conscious-sedation.

The advantages to be gained by the production of conscious-sedation must not be offset by limiting one's "technique" to specific drugs and routes of administration.

Of those routes of administration that are available for application of pharmacological agents, the following are useful for the production of conscious-sedation in dentistry:

1. Inhalation
2. Oral
3. Subcutaneous
4. Intramuscular
5. Intravenous
6. Rectal

INHALATION

The inhalation route of drug administration for the production of conscious-sedation is, for all practical purposes, limited to nitrous oxide and oxygen. This is not to say that other inhalation agents are not capable of producing similar effects. The agents that are available, however, are much more potent and are easily capable of rendering the patient unconscious. In addition, many of them possess undesirable side effects even when administered in subanesthetic doses. These factors preclude the use of all agents except nitrous oxide and oxygen for the production of conscious-sedation via the inhalation route. This route offers a pleasant and rapid method for the production of conscious-sedation, with return to the presedation state being equally rapid. Peak effectiveness will be achieved in 3 to 5 minutes. No nitrous oxide is detectable in the bloodstream 10 minutes after its inhalation is discontinued.

At times the use of this route may be of some bother, particularly when dental procedures are being carried out on maxillary anterior teeth. Various sizes and types of inhaling devices are available to aid in minimizing this inconvenience.

The inherent disadvantage of this route of administration lies with the weakness of the agent rather than the route itself. Careful preparation and selection of patients do a great deal in overcoming this disadvantage.

ORAL

Although the oral route of drug administration is the most convenient and economical, it is also the least dependable route that can be employed for the administration of conscious-sedative agents. The effectiveness of drugs administered by the oral route is influenced by many factors. The dose of the drug in question is at best an educated guess—based on the patient's age, weight, body surface area, and emotional makeup. Onset, effect, and duration are questionable because of possible destruction by digestive enzymes or combination with recently ingested food to form complexes that cannot be absorbed. When conscious-sedation is being employed, one is nearly always concerned with allaying fear and apprehension—two factors that decrease the rate of gastric emptying. The absorption of most drugs is reduced if gastric emptying is retarded. Thus the oral route of drug administration is particularly ineffective under these circumstances.

Emesis following drug ingestion, as a result of irritation to the gastrointestinal mucosa, is also a distinct possibility.

In spite of its many drawbacks the oral route is, on occasion, quite useful. When this route is chosen, one must be certain that the dose is adequate, sufficient time is allotted for drug effect, and the medication is taken when the stomach is free of recently consumed solid foods.

SUBCUTANEOUS

The subcutaneous route of drug administration may be utilized only for the administration of drugs that are not irritating to the tissues; otherwise, a slough may occur. The rate of absorption after such administration is the slowest found among the parenteral routes. Nevertheless, the route may be particularly useful when dental procedures are being carried out under regional analgesia. Certain drugs may be administered subcutaneously in the oral cavity into an area already rendered insensitive to pain. For example, a dose of atropine sufficient to decrease saliva flow may be administered into the mucobuccal fold labial to a mandibular cuspid that previously has been anesthetized with the use of an inferior alveolar nerve block. In this manner the patient is not likely to object to another needle insertion. The needle should be $1/2$ to 1 inch in length and no smaller than 25-gauge.

INTRAMUSCULAR

Drugs in aqueous solution are rapidly absorbed after deep intramuscular injection. Also those compounds too irritating to be administered by the subcutaneous route may be given via this route. Provided that the agent has been deposited deep into a large muscle mass, the rapidity of this route of injection is second only to that of the intravenous route.

Intramuscular injection sites
Lower extremity

Gluteus medius. The gluteus medius is perhaps the most commonly considered site for injections in the posterior gluteal area. Care should be exercised to restrict needle insertion to that portion of the gluteus medius muscle above an imaginary diagonal line drawn from the greater trochanter of the femur to the posterior superior iliac spine (Fig. 9-1). By administering this injection in the proper area one avoids the possibility of traumatizing the sciatic nerve or the superior gluteal artery.

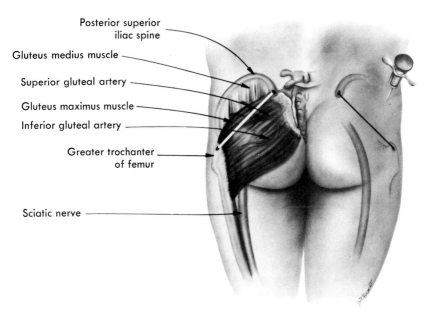

Posterior superior
iliac spine

Gluteus medius muscle

Superior gluteal artery

Gluteus maximus muscle

Inferior gluteal artery

Greater trochanter
of femur

Sciatic nerve

Fig. 9-1. Site for injection into the gluteus medius muscle.

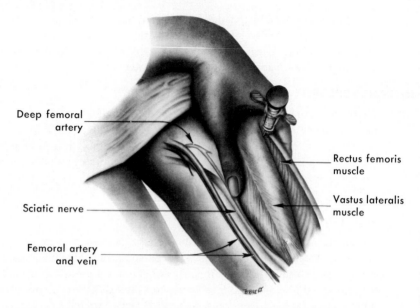

Deep femoral
artery

Rectus femoris
muscle

Vastus lateralis
muscle

Sciatic nerve

Femoral artery
and vein

Fig. 9-2. Site for injection into the vastus lateralis muscle.

The patient should lie prone in a toe-in position to relax the gluteal muscles. The needle is inserted perpendicular to the flat surface on which the patient is lying. Needle penetration should be on a direct back-to-front course.

Vastus lateralis. Another site recommended for its relative safety is the vastus lateralis. This injection is particularly well suited to children and may be administered when the patient is lying on his back or in a sitting position.

The quadriceps femoris is the largest muscle group in the anterior thigh. The vastus lateralis is the major muscle of the group and is located on the most lateral aspect of the thigh removed from major nerves and blood vessels (Fig. 9-2).

The thigh is grasped to stabilize the extremity and concentrate the muscle mass. The needle penetrates the muscle on the lateral portion of the anterior thigh and is directed in a front-to-back course. Needle penetration should not exceed 1 to 1½ inches.

Upper extremity

Mid-deltoid area. This site is frequently chosen for its ease of access and may be employed with the patient standing, seated, or recumbent.

Although the deltoid muscle forms a fairly large triangle on the shoulder prominence, the actual area of injection is limited since there are major blood vessels and nerves to be avoided.

The boundaries of injection area form a rectangle bounded by the lower

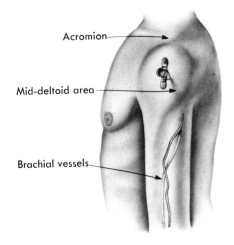

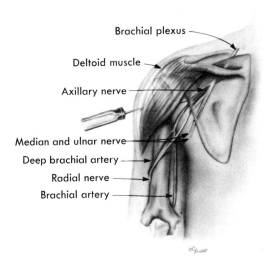

Fig. 9-3. Site for injection into the deltoid muscle.

edge of the acromion on the top to a point on the lateral side of the arm opposite the axilla on the bottom. Side boundaries are lines parallel to the arm one-third and two-thirds of the way around the outer lateral aspect of the arm (Fig. 9-3).

Injections within this area will avoid trauma to the brachial veins and arteries and the radial nerve. It is recommended that the number and size of injections made at this site be limited. The area is small and cannot tolerate repeated injections and large quantities of medications.

Technique of intramuscular injection

To carry out the intramuscular injection the following steps are performed:

1. Select the agent. When possible, select the agent that demonstrates the greatest degree of tissue tolerance.
2. Choose the appropriate injection site. In adults, the recommended site of injection is the upper outer quadrant of the gluteal area—the gluteus medius muscle. The deltoid area should be avoided in adults when anything but the most nonirritating substance is injected. In infants and children, the gluteal area is extremely small and composed mostly of fat; therefore the vastus lateralis muscle on the anterior aspect of the thigh is preferred.
3. Establish anatomic landmarks individually.
4. Cleanse the skin thoroughly with a suitable antiseptic, scrubbing in a circular fashion from the central to the peripheral zone of cleansing. Allow the antiseptic to dry before needle penetration. If an injection is made while the skin is wet, the antiseptic may be carried into the tissue, thus leading to irritation.
5. Grasp the injected site with one hand to steady the limb, tense the tissue, and compress the muscle.
6. With the syringe held in a pen grasp, with one quick thrust introduce the needle on its appropriate path. The depth of insertion varies with the individual. The needle should not be inserted to a depth exceeding three-fourths of its length.
7. Aspirate before injecting the avoid inadvertent intravascular injections.
8. Inject slowly. The solution should flow freely without force being required. The practice of extremely rapid injection, in the hope of minimizing the patient's reaction, is to be deplored. This technique usually results in the injection beginning as soon as the needle enters the skin and underlying fat and continues as the needle is advanced ("tracking"). Necrotizing lesions produced by injectables have a much greater tendency to spread in fat than in muscle. This type of technique requires that aspiration be omitted and it is highly unlikely that proper anatomic location can be achieved in such hurried procedures.
9. Use a needle of adequate length. The tendency to use a short, small gauge needle in an ill-founded attempt to minimize patient reaction is completely contrary to experimental evidence and recommended clinical procedure. The most important factor is to locate the needle tip deep within the muscle mass. Needles should be 20-gauge to 22-gauge and 1 to 2 inches in length.
10. Use disposable needles and syringes. Presterilized, disposable needles and syringes are readily available and inexpensive. The inadvertent transmission of infectious diseases is almost totally precluded.

Most injectable agents useful in the production of conscious-sedation may be administered by the intramuscular route. And, even though one must still rely on an "educated guess" for dose selection, many disadvantages inherent with the oral route are eliminated. One need not contend with enzymatic drug breakdown, the presence of food, or gastric emptying. Therefore the onset, effect, and duration of intramuscularly administered agents are rather predictable.

Most agents, when administered by this route, will be effective in 20 to 40 minutes. Variations in effect and duration will depend on the dose and pharmacological characteristics of individual compounds.

INTRAVENOUS

During the seventeenth century an artist, Christopher Wren, and a well-known chemist, Robert Boyle, combined their talents to produce one of the most important tools of medicine and dentistry, the hypodermic needle. Although their technique and device were rather crude, they were the first to produce a pharmacological effect by administering a drug directly into the bloodstream. Many advances have taken place in both technique and equipment since their crucial experiment. Today the use of the intravenous route, employing a variety of presterilized, disposable equipment, is commonplace.

Drugs in aqueous solution can be injected directly into the circulation for the production of conscious-sedation. Factors concerned with drug absorption are circumvented, and the desired blood level of the drug is obtained with an accuracy and immediacy not possible by any other route.

Drug doses may be accurately administered by delivering small aliquots and observing or "titrating" the patient to produce the desired effect. Onset will usually occur within seconds, and duration may be well controlled by selecting medications based on pharmacologically predictable traits.

The intravenous route is the method of choice when inhalation of nitrous oxide and oxygen will not suffice. Although objections are few, not all patients are amenable to intravenous medication. Patient objection or technical difficulty resulting from inaccessibility of veins, as in the obese patient, may necessitate the use of another, less desirable route.

Administration of drugs via the intravenous route is not practical in many children because of extreme emotional or behavioral difficulty. However, young age, per se, is not a contraindication to the intravenous use of drugs.

Hazards and difficulties of the intravenous route will be discussed.

Equipment

For the employment of conscious-sedation via the intravenous route a minimum amount of equipment is necessary. One should become familiar with the various types of cannulas, administration sets, etc. that are available. By having an assortment of these from which to choose one may select the equipment that best satisfies the requirements of each case.

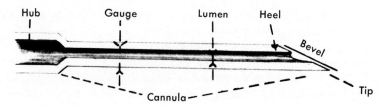

Fig. 9-4. Diagram of hollow, metal, intravenous needle. (Courtesy Abbott Laboratories.)

Types of cannulas

The hollow needle. The traditional intravenous "needle" refers to a sharpened metal cannula with a hub, by which means the skin may be penetrated and the vein entered. Usually they are made of stainless steel or aluminum and are noncorrosive and inert in relation to tissues. The hollow needle consists of a hub, shaft (or cannula), and bevel. (See Fig. 9-4.)

The bevel of a hollow needle may be any one of three types: the single, a variation of the single, and the triple. Initially, intravenous hollow needles were of the single-bevel variety; that is, only one "grind" was performed in the tip of the cannula to yield the finished product. This resulted in the production of an extremely long bevel if one was to have a needle with a gradual taper. The excessive length of the bevel was prone to penetrate the opposite side of the vessel during venipuncture, particularly when small veins were being cannulated. Variations of this needle led to the development of the triple-bevel needle. With this needle all angles or grinds must complement each other so that resistance while entering the vein is minimized.

The term "gauge" refers to the caliber of the cannula of a needle. Currently needles that are marked "intravenous" range from 14-gauge to 25-gauge. The larger the gauge number, the smaller the lumen size. Needles of high gauge numbers are suitable for entering small veins or for administering solutions of low viscosity (Fig. 9-5).

The length, together with the gauge of the needle, usually determines what the type of the needle is and where it is to be used; a short needle is regarded as convenient when entering small veins, but a long needle is preferred when percutaneous venipuncture of larger veins of the forearm is being performed.

The factor of disposability is also important when considering needles for venipuncture. Formerly, the needle would be resharpened and resterilized between applications. Often rough edges remained on the needle, resulting in excessive damage at the site of venipuncture. Current needle design is based on the premise that the needle is truly sharp only once and that each sub-

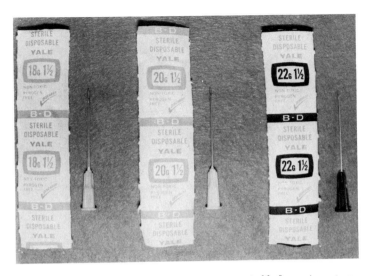

Fig. 9-5. Disposable metal needles, various sizes, suitable for venipuncture.

sequent use of the needle results in undue trauma to the patient undergoing venipuncture.

Some needles are coated with silicone during the manufacturing process. This reduces the amount of friction between tissue and needle during insertion and allows the needle to slide more smoothly into the vein. Siliconized needles are also "hemorepellent," which means that clot formation within the needle is less likely to occur.

Many modern needles are designated as "thinwall." This term implies that the wall is thinner than the standard needle and offers the advantage of a larger internal diameter for the particular external diameter and thus the possibility of higher flow rates.

The hollow needle most popular today may be siliconized, has a triple bevel, must be sharp and noncorrosive, should be both disposable and available in a variety of sizes to meet technical requirements of various venipuncture procedures.

Winged needles. The most widespread derivation of the plain hollow needle currently available is the winged infusion set (Fig. 9-6, *A*). Needles of this type are regarded by many to be the needle of choice for venipuncture of superficial veins in patients of all ages.

The winged infusion set consists of a stainless steel needle, two flexible wing-like plastic projections mounted to the shank of the needle, a variable length of flexible tubing, and a female Luer adapter that accepts any standard infusion set. The wings serve as a convenient grip during insertion and allow for secure taping after venipuncture has been completed. (See Fig. 9-6, *B* and

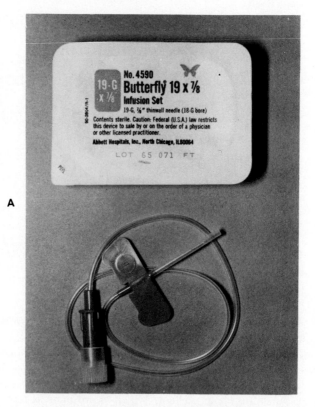

A

Fig. 9-6. A, A 19-gauge winged needle. **B,** Grasp employed for insertion of winged needle. **C,** Winged needle taped in place.

C.) This short-beveled, short-shafted needle is particularly useful when the patient is to be positioned in a dental chair.

Catheter-over-needle units. Modern plastic catheter-over-needle devices (Fig. 9-7) have overcome the two technical problems initially associated with their designs: (1) devising a suitable initial taper, to ease catheter insertion, and (2) firmly bonding the catheter to the hub.

Catheter insertion has also been facilitated by using a material such as Teflon and manufacturing it of radiopaque components permits better visualization radiographically in the event that the catheter is inadvertently severed and migrates from the site of injection.

Regardless of the particular design employed, the procedure for insertion of the catheter-over-needle device is the same. The catheter accompanies the needle into the vein during venipuncture. Once in the vein the needle is withdrawn, allowing the catheter, which is connected to the infusion set, to remain.

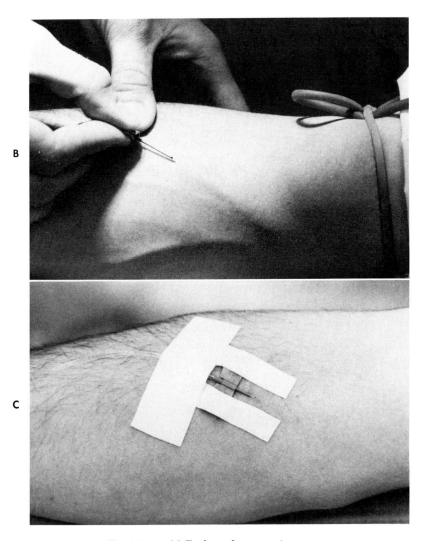

Fig. 9-6, cont'd. For legend see opposite page.

Because the catheter is pliable and contains no sharp needle bevel, the incidence of potential complications is reduced.

The catheter-over-needle unit is particularly useful for patients seated in a dental chair. Its flexibility allows placement in the dorsum of the hand, the wrist, or antecubital fossa and does not require restraint or the use of an arm board. Once positioned, the patient may assume a comfortable position, and movement of the arm is relatively unrestricted.

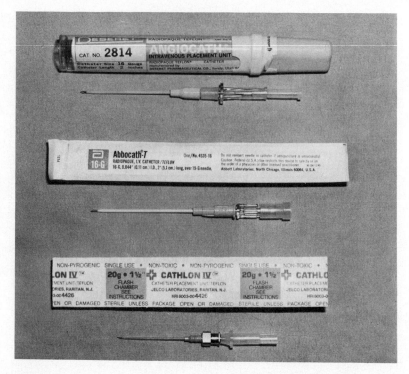

Fig. 9-7. Catheter-over-needle units. Top to bottom: Angiocath, Abbocath, Jelco Cathlon IV.

Administration sets and solutions

The administration set and intravenous solution should be utilized for the convenience of the dentist and the comfort of the patient (Fig. 9-8). If a solution of 5% dextrose in water, normal saline, or lactated Ringer's solution in 5% dextrose is infused at a very slow rate, the cannula will remain patent throughout the conscious-sedative procedure. All medications may be given into the injection site on the administration set, thereby eliminating the need for subsequent venipuncture or troublesome replacement of a syringe that is attached to the venous cannula.

Supplementary drugs may be administered as required throughout management of the case; in the event that an emergency occurs, requiring the use of drugs, these may be readily administered via the intravenous infusion.

A properly placed intravenous infusion will not cause the patient any discomfort, and it provides a convenience for the dentist that aids in the smooth course of the conscious-sedative experience.

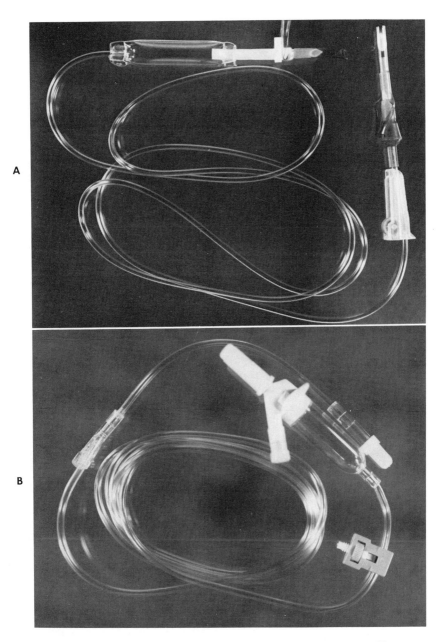

Fig. 9-8. Administration sets. **A,** With rubber injection site. **B,** Without rubber injection site.   *Continued.*

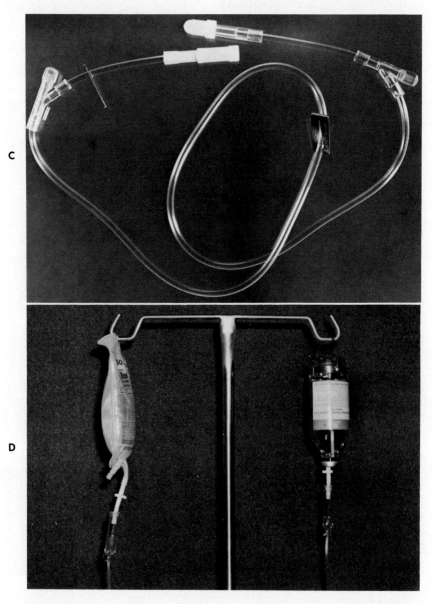

Fig. 9-8, cont'd. C, Secondary administration set with two injection sites. **D,** Stand, used in giving 5% dextrose in water solutions, with administration sets attached.

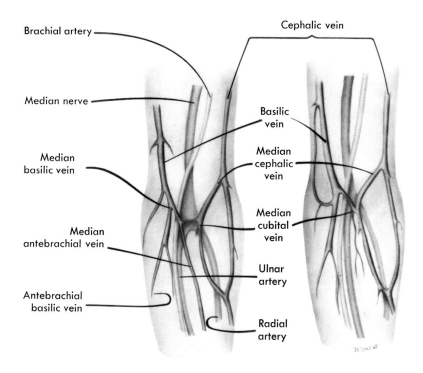

Fig. 9-9. Relationship of superficial arteries, veins, and nerves, illustrated by two common vein arrangements in the antecubital fossa of the left arm.

Venipuncture technique
Selecting and preparing the site for injection

If the venipuncture is to be as safe and painless as possible, certain preliminary precautions should be observed. Although most superficial veins are suitable for venipuncture, veins in the antecubital fossa (median basilic and median cephalic) are most frequently chosen because they are usually large and easily accessible. (See Fig. 9-9.) However, this site is not the best in all instances. Other alternatives are available, sometimes with advantage. One must also bear in mind the fact that the median nerve lies in the antecubital fossa and that, in some patients, the brachial artery may lie superficially. Prior to application of a tourniquet and venipuncture the brachial artery should be located by palpation, so that it may be avoided during needle insertion (Fig. 9-10).

Other available veins include the cephalic and basilic veins in the arm above the antecubital fossa and veins in the metacarpal and dorsal venous network on the back of the hand (Fig. 9-11). The accessory cephalic and median antebrachial veins of the forearm are favored by many dentists because

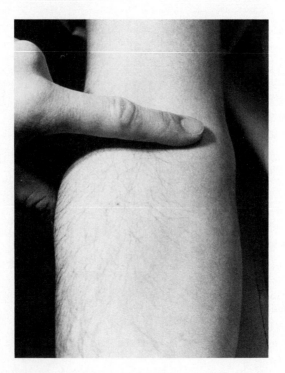

Fig. 9-10. Palpation of brachial artery of the right arm prior to venipuncture in ante-cubital fossa.

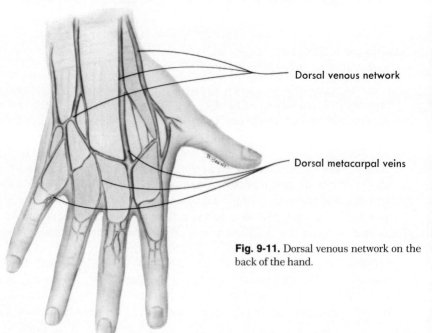

Dorsal venous network

Dorsal metacarpal veins

Fig. 9-11. Dorsal venous network on the back of the hand.

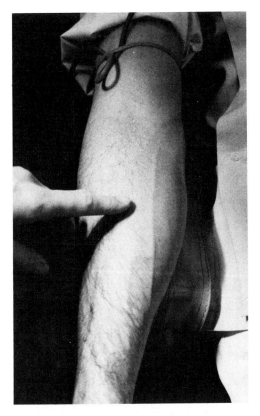

Fig. 9-12. Accessory cephalic and median antebrachial veins of the forearm are well suited for venipuncture.

they are usually accessible and are rather straight and fixed in position so that minor arm movement is not likely to dislodge the cannula or cause it to penetrate the posterior wall of the vessel. (See Fig. 9-12.)

Once the site for venipuncture has been selected, utmost care should be directed toward proper distention of the vein. As a simple preliminary measure, the arm in which the vein is located should be allowed to hang dependent for a time. This maneuver will allow the veins to become more apparent.

For those veins that stand out well, mild manual compression above the site with a tourniquet will be sufficient to fill them. The tourniquet should be applied on the upper arm above the antecubital fossa and be tightened sufficiently to obstruct venous outflow without hindering arterial inflow. After the tourniquet is applied, the patient should be instructed to continually open and close his hand, finally keeping it closed until the cannula is positioned in the vein.

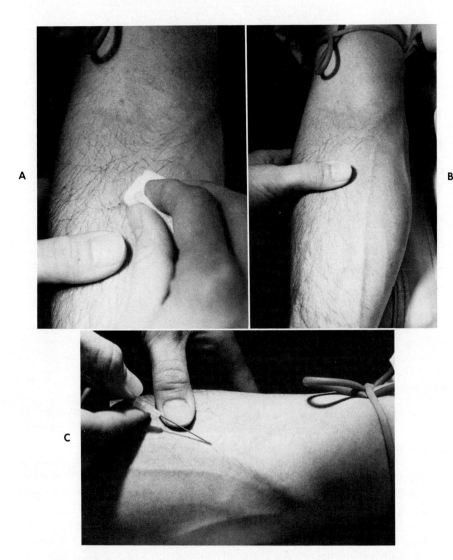

Fig. 9-13. A, Suitable antiseptic solution is applied to the site prior to venipuncture. **B,** Arm is held by the operator's left hand to tense the skin and stabilize the vein. **C,** Needle enters skin at 45-degree angle to the surface. **D,** Needle pierces skin and underlying tissue down to depth of vein. **E,** Angle of needle is decreased and advanced into the vein. **F,** Vein is gently lifted on the needle as it is advanced into vein.

In general, the larger the vessel in relation to the gauge of the cannula, the less the likelihood that irritation will occur. This is due to the fact that the fluid being administered is likely to undergo more rapid dilution in the bloodstream when the caliber of the vein exceeds the outside diameter of the cannula. There is also less chance of foreign body reaction when the cannula does not come in contact with the vessel wall.

Making the venipuncture

After the vein has been selected, an arm board may facilitate the puncture by preventing the patient from moving his arm.

The area over the puncture site should be cleansed with a suitable antiseptic prior to needle insertion. Some investigators consider it important to use both a defatting agent and an antibacterial agent. Some individuals use 70% isopropyl alcohol, whereas others prefer benzalkonium chloride tincture and 70% alcohol solution, 99% isopropyl alcohol, and povidone-iodine (Betadine). Sterile tape or occlusive dressings would be applied to the site after venipuncture is completed to secure the cannula in position.

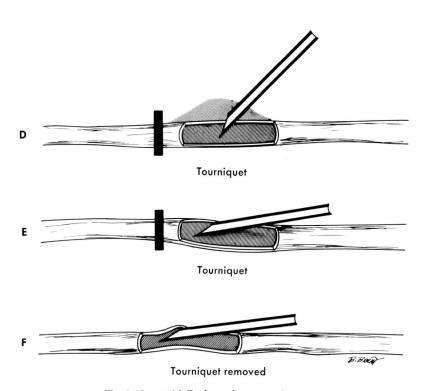

D

Tourniquet

E

Tourniquet

F

Tourniquet removed

Fig. 9-13, cont'd. For legend see opposite page.

After selecting and distending the vein and preparing the site of insertion the venipuncture proceeds with these basic steps:

1. Apply antiseptic solution to injection site (Fig. 9-13, *A*).
2. Clear infusion tubing of air and fasten pinch clamp.
3. Hold the arm with the left hand, using the thumb to place the skin on stretch and anchor in vein (Fig. 9-13, *B*).
4. Point the needle in the direction of the course of the vein at the proposed site of entry. The angle of the needle to the surface should be about 45 degrees and the bevel facing upward (Fig. 9-13, *C*).
5. Place the tip of the needle slightly to one side of the vein and about $1/2$ inch below the point where the needle will enter the vein itself.
6. Firmly pierce the skin and underlying tissues to the depth of the vein (Fig. 9-13, *D*).
7. Depress the needle (decrease its angle) so that the needle is almost flush with the skin. Move the tip of the needle directly above the vein.
8. Slowly push the needle into the vein (Fig. 9-13, *E*). A backflow of blood into the clear plastic tubing will indicate satisfactory entry.

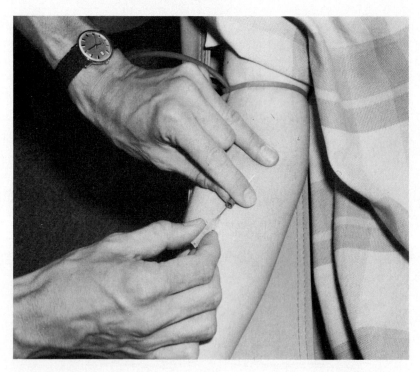

Fig. 9-14. Third finger of left hand occludes tip of cannula while thumb and index finger of right hand steady hub for withdrawal of metal needle and attachment of administration set.

9. When the blood appears, cautiously advance the needle until it lies well within the lumen of the vein. This should be done by gently lifting the vein on the needle with a slight upward pressure to prevent the needle's passing through the posterior wall of the vein. (See Fig. 9-13, *F.*)

10. Release the tourniquet and relax the tension on the skin.

11. Adjust pinch clamp and start the infusion.

12. Examine the site to be sure fluid is flowing freely in the vein. Swelling may indicate extravasation. In this event, the infusion should be discontinued immediately and a new site selected.

13. Tape the needle firmly in place.

The technique is altered slightly when catheter-over-needle units are employed. After the needle carries the catheter into the vein (step 8), the unit is advanced a very short distance. The third finger of the left hand applies pressure over the tip of the catheter while the thumb and index finger grasp the hub of the catheter. (See Fig. 9-14.) The tourniquet is removed and the needle is then withdrawn and discarded, an infusion set is attached and turned on, and the catheter is slowly advanced into position, then taped securely.

This maneuver allows for easy venipuncture and prevents blood from leaking from the catheter as the needle is withdrawn and the infusion started. By starting the infusion before advancing the catheter the infusion liquid "lubricates" the vessel and tends to make catheter insertion easier and less traumatic.

Discontinuing the infusion

At the completion of the infusion attention must be paid to proper technique for discontinuing the infusion, according to the following sequence:

1. Shut the pinch clamp to stop the infusion.

2. Release all tape securing the cannula.

3. Place a sterile piece of cotton over the puncture site and gently withdraw the cannula. *Do not* apply pressure at this time, lest the cannula irritate the vein and result in a local reaction.

4. Apply and maintain pressure over the puncture site for 30 to 60 seconds following cannula removal.

5. Apply a topical antibiotic ointment to the puncture site and cover with a sterile dressing.

Venipuncture complications

Intravenous procedures carry certain risks or hazards to the patient. Fortunately, most if not all of these are preventable by adherence to established principles and previously described precautionary measures. Indeed, the increasing frequency with which intravenous procedures are used attests to the wide recognition of their safety. Problems associated with venipuncture can be divided into local reactions and systemic complications.

Local reactions at or near the site of venipuncture

Nonvenous. The most commonly encountered sequela of venipuncture is the small painless hematoma of the puncture wound. It may vary in size and may be minimized by compression at the puncture site with sterile cotton when the needle is withdrawn. It is caused by the minor trauma of skin penetration. A slightly greater reaction may result in a painful hematoma with some residual tenderness. A more diffuse reaction of this kind is accompanied by edema and some reddening at the site of needle entry but does not involve the vein. These complications usually resolve without treatment. Very infrequently these degrees of reaction involve cellulitis or suppuration.

Venous. In addition to the foregoing nonvenous reactions, less common but more severe local reactions may involve the vein at or near the site of venipuncture. These reactions may be classified as follows:

1. *Thrombosis* — painless or slightly tender thrombus (clot) develops in the area of cannula entry after cannula's removal.

2. *Phlebitis* — pain, usually severe, occurs at the site of cannula entry and extends for a variable distance along the vein, sometimes the length of the arm, accompanied by acute tenderness, redness, and slight edema of the vein; the condition worsens if infusion is continued or rate increased but usually subsides if infusion is stopped; thrombophlebitis may develop. Local application of heat will relieve discomfort.

3. *Thrombophlebitis* — thrombus formation preceded by phlebitis as above (severity is determined by length of vein involved), often accompanied by fever, malaise, and leukocytosis. Acute symptoms usually subside in a very few days, but tenderness may persist for several weeks, eventually leaving a firm, painless, cord-like vein, with or without brown or green discoloration of the overlying skin. Suppuration is uncommon, but systemic thrombophlebitis may occur with serious consequences.

Factors involved in local reactions

Precise information is lacking regarding the incidence or cause of local reactions. There is some evidence to indicate that the incidence of local reactions increases with the duration of the infusion, but it is not established that the severity of local complications increases with infusion time.

The following factors have been considered as potential causes of local reactions: pH of infusate; components of infusate; rate and duration of infusion; mechanical factors (bevel and dullness of needle, technique, etc.); size of needle in relation to caliber of vein; pressure of injection; disease, age, and sex of the patient.

The underlying causes of local vein reactions have yet to be completely elucidated. Although infection, when present, constitutes an etiological basis, the majority of local complications have not been attributed to the entry of

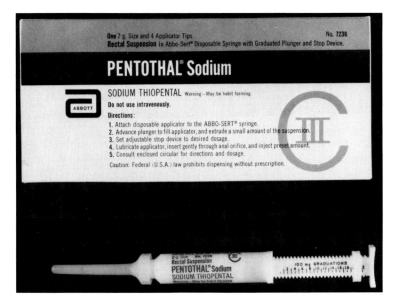

Fig. 9-15. Rectal thiopental (Pentothal) preparation. (Courtesy Abbott Laboratories.)

pathogenic microorganisms. Some authorities are more inclined to relate the occurrence of local effects to chemical irritation from drugs or infusates or from foreign body reactions.

Systemic complications

Although systemic complications such as septicemia or catheter and air embolisms may be attributed to venous cannulation and intravenous fluid administration, their occurrence is strictly limited to long-term therapy. Description of these complications need not be included in a discussion involving intravenous infusions of relatively brief duration.

RECTAL

The rectal route of drug administration is particularly useful for uncooperative children. A state of conscious-sedation may usually be achieved in 8 to 10 minutes. However, drug absorption via this route may be irregular and incomplete, thus decreasing the predictability of drug onset and effect.

The most popular agent for the production of conscious-sedation via the rectal route is thiopental (Fig. 9-15). For the production of conscious-sedation an average dose is 1 gm. of thiopental for each 50 to 75 pounds of body weight (10 to 13.5 mg. per pound).

SUMMARY

The technical methods required for administration of drugs by various routes have been presented, as well as their advantages and disadvantages. The practitioner should familiarize himself with all routes of administration and employ the appropriate method when indicated.

One must bear in mind that the route of administration is only as safe as the practitioner who uses it. It must be stressed that, regardless of the choice of drug or its route of administration, once medication has been administered the patient must remain under constant surveillance throughout his stay in the dental office. It is the dentist's obligation to safeguard the life and welfare of his patient throughout the course of dental treatment.

Chapter 10

TECHNIQUE FOR INTRAVENOUS CONSCIOUS-SEDATION

For conscious-sedation via the intravenous route to be successful all parameters discussed in previous chapters must be integrated in a well-organized "plan of attack." Difficulties that may be encountered should be anticipated so that necessary steps may be taken to avoid them if possible. Appointments must be so structured that a maximum amount of efficiently delivered dental health care may be accomplished while the patient is in a comfortable, apprehension-free and pain-free state.

INITIAL PATIENT VISIT

Although the fact is not fully appreciated by many practitioners, patient-dentist relationship actually starts long *before* the patient confronts the practitioner in the dental office. Similarly, the patient does not begin to *seek* dental care with the first office visit. Patient-dentist relationships as well as the seeking of dental care begin with the patient's first inquiry of friends, relatives, etc. as to which dentist in the area should be consulted regarding dental services. Few patients will select a dentist at random. They would much rather be referred to a practitioner by one who has been treated himself.

Thus the patient presenting in a dental office for the first time arrives with preconceived notions regarding the practitioner as well as his office and auxiliary personnel. If the patient's "set" concerning the office is favorable, the patient-dentist relationship is more likely to be satisfactory than if the patient's attitude is unfavorable.

Even though the practitioner may not have had previous contact with a particular patient, he may be able to influence the attitude of the patient before he enters the office. This may be accomplished by properly managing the patients currently undergoing dental treatment, who in future times will be the individuals to either recommend or discourage treatment in a particular office.

It is imperative, therefore, that the practitioner be as thorough and understanding as possible of the needs of each individual patient. Not only will the patient benefit from the care and consideration being extended but also the practitioner stands to gain from the reputation he is establishing.

On occasion patients will present for dental treatment, having misconceptions about dental care rendered with the aid of conscious-sedation. All misunderstandings must be clarified prior to the start of treatment—for the benefit of patient and dentist alike.

Patient evaluation

At the initial visit the dentist must attempt to establish good patient rapport by demonstrating his concern for the problems presented. The medical and dental histories should be taken by the dentist himself to aid in establishing a favorable relationship, to give the patient an opportunity to express himself to the dentist, and to better enable the clinician to evaluate the physical and psychological condition of the patient. The more thorough the history, the more useful will be the information gained. The physical examination should also be carried out by the dentist, since he can thus better correlate the findings with historical information.

Primary goals of the pretreatment evaluation are to allow the dentist to assess the physical and psychological conditions of the patient, to select those patients who because of impaired conditions are prime candidates for conscious-sedation, and to identify the "awareness level" of his patient, that he may better choose the conscious-sedative technique that best fulfills the needs of the individual.

After the pretreatment evaluation a thorough dental examination should be completed. This examination must also be as thorough as possible and on occasion should be accomplished at a subsequent appointment, with the aid of conscious-sedation. For the dental examination to be most useful in formulation of a treatment plan, it should be completed under as nearly ideal conditions as possible. The pretreatment evaluation and the dental examination will go hand in hand when the dentist is deciding on the treatment regimen to be followed throughout the case.

By combining information gained from these examinations one is better able to determine the requirements of the conscious-sedative technique from both the patient's and the practitioner's point of view. Taking into account the type of dental work required and the time necessary to perform it coupled with the patient's overall condition will allow for the most judicious use of chair time—for patient and dentist. The number of appointments and their approximate duration should be estimated, since this information will aid in the selection of intravenous drugs.

Case presentation

Once the entire treatment plan has been formulated and the need and usefulness of conscious-sedation established, the case should be presented to the patient. The amount and types of dental services as well as the time required should be explained to the patient along with the advantages to be gained through the use of conscious-sedation.

The patient should be told that medication will be administered intravenously to place him in such a condition that he is relaxed, comfortable, and somewhat sleepy, yet conscious and aware of his surroundings at all times. He should be informed that, although conscious, he will have an indifferent attitude toward the dental procedure, will be free of all discomfort, may not have a clear recollection of the appointment, and will not realize the passage of time at a normal rate. Hence, a greater amount of dental treatment can be more efficiently rendered when conscious-sedation is employed, eliminating the need for frequent visits to the dental office.

Emphasis should be placed on the fact that conscious-sedation and general anesthesia are not the same entity. Some individuals having fears related to the unconscious state must have their fears dispelled with a clear explanation of conscious-sedation. Others who state a preference to be "completely out" must have the advantages of conscious-sedation over general anesthesia enumerated.

A few patients have the misconception that unless they are unconscious they will be able to feel pain during dental operations. This wrongful impression may be a previous, unpleasant dental experience or by the fact that other dental procedures were carried out under general anesthesia. The patient must be assured that, with this modality, pain-free dentistry is easily accomplished and that if at any time he experiences discomfort all he need do is report it and it will promptly be controlled.

An occasional patient will express concern over the fact that he "might talk" or divulge secrets while under the influence of conscious-sedation. This fear is unfounded, and the patient must be assured that such is not the case. He is no more likely to divulge secrets while under conscious-sedation than in his present state, since he will remain conscious throughout the procedure. Unless the patient expresses a fear of divulging secrets, no mention should be made of it lest the seed of this fear be planted in the patient's mind.

Prior to arranging for subsequent appointments and the use of conscious-sedation the patient should be instructed in and given procedures to be followed on the day of the next appointment. A written copy of the instructions should be given to the patient as well, to be certain that all confusion is eliminated. The instructions should include the following information:

1. The last meal that is eaten prior to the appointment should be eaten about 2 to 2$^{1}/_{2}$ hours before the scheduled appointment time. It should consist of light liquids such as broth, tea, and gelatin dessert. (Although having a full stomach is not hazardous when conscious-sedation is employed, it tends to increase the incidence of nausea and vomiting, which are unpleasant at best.)

2. Clothes worn at the appointment should be loose fitting and comfortable, preferably short sleeved.

3. Since the patient may be a bit drowsy on dismissal and may have minor sensory imbalances, for his safety he *must* be escorted from the office by a responsible adult.

4. The patient should be cautioned against sitting up or standing suddenly after the appointment. This may lead to transient dizzy spells. Changing position slowly will eliminate this side effect.

5. Following the patient's dismissal, mild sleepiness may persist for a brief period of time. A short nap for an hour or so is recommended.

6. Warn the patient, for his safety, not to engage in any activity that requires sensory and motor coordination during the following 24 hours. Such activities as driving an automobile or operating power tools are forbidden during this period.

7. The patient should not indulge in any alcoholic beverages for 24 hours after the conscious-sedative procedure. Alcohol is capable of potentiating many agents used for conscious-sedation.

Having examined, selected, and prepared the patient physically and psychologically and having formulated the total treatment plan, the dentist is ready to extend dental services with the aid of conscious-sedation.

DENTAL TREATMENT WITH CONSCIOUS-SEDATION
Selection of agents and equipment

On the basis of the medical, psychological, and dental findings acquired during the initial visit the dentist is prepared to select the pharmacological agents to be employed in the conscious-sedative technique.

Drug selection should be based on the following factors:

1. *Conscious-sedative effect required.* If identical effects are to be achieved, those patients having a very apprehensive "level of awareness" will require more potent agents than those with a moderate or mild level.

2. *Need for the production of amnesia.* Patients who have expressed a fear related to a particular aspect of dental treatment, such as application of regional analgesia, will fare better if drugs are included that provide a degree of amnesia.

3. *Necessity of including a narcotic analgetic.* The desirability of including drugs that elevate the pain threshold in addition to allaying fear and apprehension must be ascertained. This is best done by first, determining the probability that one will secure adequate regional analgesia and, second, considering the length of the appointment. In a certain few patients one will have difficulty in securing profound regional analgesia. This may be caused by physical characteristics of the patient, such as obesity or anatomical variations. When difficulty is expected, a narcotic analgetic should be employed to aid in pain control by its action on the central nervous system. In other cases in which an extended period of time has been allotted for the procedure, patients usually fare better when a narcotic analgetic is employed even though adequate regional analgesia is easily accomplished. With inclusion of these drugs minor annoyances unrelated to the operative site are better tolerated. For example, discomfort in the temporomandibular joint and related structures, which is associated with prolonged mouth opening, is easily eliminated.

4. *Duration for which the effect is required.* For those cases that are to be brief duration drugs with the shortest effect are to be chosen. Longer cases will require the judicious selection of those agents having appropriate durations. The necessity of narcotic analgetics in cases of more than brief duration was discussed before.

5. *Special conditions of the patient.* Special conditions with which the patient may present militate against the use of certain drugs. A history of an allergic reaction, for example, may preclude the use of some agents, and the presence of porphyria may make the selection of barbiturates unwise. After having selected and readied the agents that will best fill the requirements of patient and dentist, the appropriate administration set, intravenous fluid, and intravenous cannula should be assembled. All accessory equipment such as tape and gauze sponges should be on hand and within easy reach.

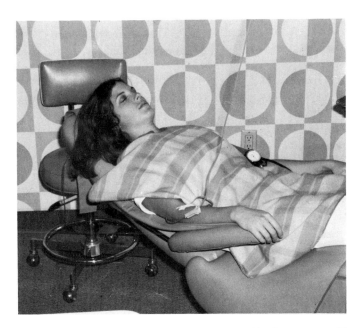

Fig. 10-1. Patient seated in contour dental chair, with blood pressure cuff and intravenous infusion in place.

Chairside procedure

The patient is seated comfortably in the dental chair, which is then tilted backward, placing the patient in a semireclining position. (Although not a requirement, a contour-type dental chair is ideally suited for dentistry with conscious-sedation.) Placing the patient in this position permits maximum comfort for both patient and operator. The position also aids normal physiological function of the patient's cardiovascular and respiratory systems. Venous return is facilitated, both decreasing the possibility of a bout of psychologically induced syncope and reducing the chance of drug-induced hypotension. Simultaneously, normal respiratory system function is maintained, since the abdominal viscera do not interfere with normal diaphragmatic movement. A blood pressure cuff is placed on the patient's left arm and the initial blood pressure measurement is taken and recorded. Likewise, pulse rate and rhythm and the respiratory rate, depth, and character are noted and recorded. In most apprehensive patients these values will be slightly above those obtained while the individual is at rest. After examination of the right arm and hand and selection of a convenient site for venipuncture, an intravenous infusion of 5% dextrose in water is started. Intravenous drugs employed in the conscious-sedative technique are administered into the injection site of the administration set. (See Fig. 10-1.)

Psychosedative administration

It is my belief that when several drugs are being employed in the conscious-sedative technique one should administer the psychosedative agent first. Such drugs generally have a minimal effect when given alone and are rather slow in onset, but they have the ability to potentiate other agents that are to follow in sequence. By administering the psychosedative agent first one may more effectively titrate the minimal dosage of narcotic analgetics and barbiturates to their desired effect. Incremental doses are administered at 30- to 45-second intervals until the desired effect is achieved. The patient will become calmed and nervous mannerisms tend to subside. Reports of mild sleep-

Table 3. Characteristics of psychosedative agents

Drug	I.V. dose	Comment
Promethazine (Phenergan)	25 to 50 mg.	Produces little sedation; good potentiating ability
Propiomazine (Largon)	10 to 20 mg.	Similar to promethazine
Diazepam (Valium)	5 to 15 mg.	Produces good calming effect; good potentiating ability; amnesic qualities; must not be diluted—given directly into I.V. cannula

iness or a heavy, relaxed feeling are not uncommon and the patient may have difficulty keeping the eyes open. Pulse rate and blood pressure may be somewhat lower than presedative levels, because of the calming effect manifested. Those patients who exhibit a very mild degree of apprehension may be satisfactorily managed with a psychosedative agent alone.

Many psychosedative drugs are available, but the agents listed in Table 3 have been found to be particularly useful.

Most psychosedative drugs will have a duration of about 1 to 1½ hours after intravenous injection of the recommended dose.

Narcotic analgetic administration

For those individual judged to be moderately apprehensive, a combination of a psychosedative plus a narcotic analgetic may be desirable. After production of a "background" effect through administration of the psychosedative agent the overall effect may be further enhanced by adding incremental doses of narcotic analgetics. As this drug effect is realized, the patient becomes more relaxed and calmed. He reports symptoms related to the euphoric state. A pleasant smile may come over his face and he will report that he feels "great" when questioned. It is not uncommon for patients to state that they "would not mind feeling this good all of the time," that they "have not been this relaxed in weeks," or that they are "totally indifferent" toward the scheduled dental procedure.

In contrast to the psychosedative agents, there are several narcotic analgetic drugs available that possess varying durations. The agents in Table 4 are a few of the narcotic analgetics that have been shown to be useful in conscious-sedation.

As indicated in Table 4, the narcotic analgetics may be used either alone or in combination with psychosedative agents to produce similar effects. However, when used alone, greater doses are required.

Barbiturate administration

Although the barbiturates have the ability to lower the pain reaction threshold and decrease the patient's ability to tolerate pain, they are very valuable agents for the production of conscious-sedation, particularly if regional analgesia is easily secured. They may be used alone for the production of conscious-sedation or in combination with psychosedatives and narcotic analgetics.

When they are used in conjunction with other agents, it is my belief that the barbiturates should be administered last in the sequence. They, like the narcotic analgetics, are potentiated by the psychosedative agents. Their onset is more rapid than that of either the psychosedative or the narcotic analgetic and, if the ultrashort barbiturates are chosen, they are more potent than either of the other two agents. In the presence of narcotic analgetics the barbiturates

Table 4. Characteristics of narcotic analgetic agents

Drug	I.V. dose alone	Dose with psychosedative	Duration	Comment
Meperidine (Demerol)	50 to 100 mg.	25 to 50 mg.	1 to 1½ hours	Good analgesia; good calming and euphoric qualities
Anileridine (Leritine)	25 to 50 mg.	10 to 25 mg.	1 to 1½ hours	Similar to meperidine
Morphine	10 to 15 mg.	3 to 10 mg.	2 to 2½ hours	Good analgesia; good calming and euphoric qualities
Alphaprodine (Nisentil)	40 to 60 mg.	20 to 30 mg.	30 to 45 minutes	Similar to meperidine
Fentanyl (Sublimaze)	0.1 to 0.25 mg.	0.05 to 0.15 mg.	30 minutes	Good analgesia; poor calming and euphoric qualities

Table 5. Characteristics of barbiturate sedative-hypnotics

Drug	Dose alone	Dose with psychosedative and narcotic analgetic	Duration	Comment
Methohexital (Brevital)	20 to 40 mg.	5 to 20 mg.	5 to 10 minutes	Good sedation; good amnesia; most potent barbiturate
Pentobarbital (Nembutal)	50 to 100 mg.	25 to 50 mg.	1½ to 2 hours	Good sedative effects; longest-acting I.V. agent
Thiopental (Pentothal) or thiamylal (Surital)	50 to 100 mg.	25 to 50 mg.	20 to 40 minutes	Good sedative effects; short-duration I.V. agents

also have a greater sedative effect, thus allowing smaller doses to be employed.

Therefore one administers the drug with the mildest effect first and the one with the most intense effect and most rapid onset last. In this manner one is not likely to "overshoot" the mark and administer a greater dose of any one agent than is required.

When barbiturates are combined with other agents they add a degree of sedation, sleepiness, and amnesia not possible with other agents.

The characteristics of some of the most popular barbiturates are listed in Table 5.

Of these agents methohexital is the most popular, since its duration is the shortest. One can easily administer additional increments as required to sustain its effect. It has particularly good amnesic qualities in the conscious patient. One must bear in mind, however, that the ultrashort barbiturates (methohexital, thiopental, and thiamylal) are extremely potent, and the recommended dose must be administered in very small increments while the patient is observed for drug effects. The same total dose administered in a bolus is likely to render the patient unconscious, a potentially dangerous situation.

After having administered both the psychosedative and the narcotic analgetics, one may administer methohexital in 5 mg. (0.5 ml.) increments every 30 to 45 seconds until the patient relates the presence of a definite sleepy or groggy sensation. He will become even more relaxed than before, speech will become slurred, and he may have difficulty focusing his eyes.

At this point the patient will be calmed, have a freedom from fear and apprehension, be sedate or sleepy, and be in an amnesic state that will last about 10 minutes. During this period one may perform those necessary but particularly bothersome procedures such as the production of regional analgesia. Although at this point the patient is in a calmed and care-free state, he may react to mildly painful stimuli (for example, regional analgesia production) with a facial grimace or a movement. Nevertheless he is capable of rational response to command (such as "open your mouth") at all times. One must not attempt to eliminate the reaction to painful stimuli by increasing the dose of the barbiturate. To accomplish this, the patient must be rendered unconscious.

Although the barbiturates may be used alone for the production of conscious-sedation, their primary advantage lies in their ability to complement the psychosedatives and narcotic analgetics. When used alone they will sometimes make the patient less, rather than more, cooperative. Since their solitary use lowers the pain threshold, one must be particularly careful to avoid any painful stimulation under these circumstances.

Care must be used when employing the barbiturates and narcotic analgetics in combination or sequence. Because of the pH of these agents they will precipitate if mixed in the same syringe. If one agent is administered immediately after the other into the injection site of an intravenous infusion, a sufficient amount of infusate should be allowed to wash the line clear before the next agent is administered, lest precipitation occur within the tubing of the administration set.

Belladonna administration

The administration of atropine or scopolamine may occur at any time after the intravenous infusion is started. The belladonna drugs may be mixed in the same syringe with any agent(s) (except diazepam) used for the production of conscious-sedation. They will have their peak effect on decreasing the flow of saliva in 2 to 5 minutes and will be effective for 1 to 1^1/$_2$ hours. Since some of the other agents used for the production of conscious-sedation also have the ability to decrease the flow of saliva, belladonna drugs are not required routinely. Their use should be restricted to those cases in which excessive saliva creates a bothersome environment for dental procedures. *The use of scopolamine is not recommended in outpatients.*

• • •

As the intravenous medication is administered, the dentist's free hand should palpate the radial pulse to note changes in its rate. As a calming effect comes over the patient, the pulse rate and blood pressure usually fall from their previously elevated levels to within normal limits. Because of the maintenance of normal physiological function, vital signs will not be depressed below these limits. That is to say that one will rarely, if ever, observe hypotension or bradycardia. After the patient has been placed in a satisfactory state of conscious-sedation, the pulse rate and blood pressure are noted and regional analgesia is secured.

Securing regional analgesia

Following the administration of all intravenous agents that are required to place the patient in the desired state of conscious-sedation, regional analgesia is secured in the usual manner. The use of a topical antiseptic and a topical anesthetic solution is strongly recommended.

All areas to be involved in dental procedures may be anesthetized at this time, or the dentist may prefer to anesthetize one quadrant or one arch at a time. From a safety point of view, all areas of the oral cavity may satisfactorily be anesthetized simultaneously, since no protective reflexes are obtunded by this maneuver. However, at the completion of the appointment, having the entire oral cavity anesthetized may be bothersome or uncomfortable to the patient. Inadvertent trauma to soft tissues while talking may also occur.

At this point it is extremely important to reiterate the necessity for profound regional analgesia for the control of operative pain during conscious-sedation. If the conscious-sedative procedure is less than satisfactory, one must first consider the possibility that regional analgesia is inadequate. *The*

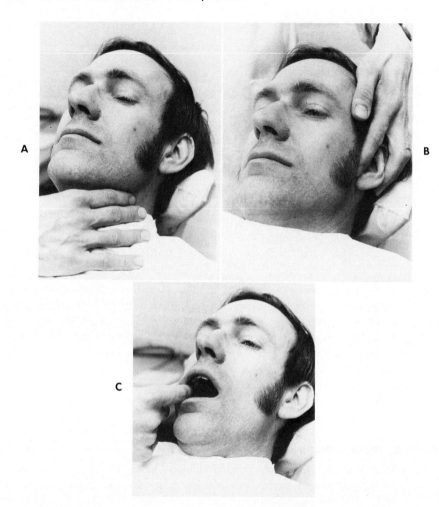

Fig. 10-2. Palpation of arteries. **A,** Carotid artery. **B,** Superficial temporal artery. **C,** Facial artery in the cheek.

key to the success of conscious-sedation is proper control of operative pain through the use of regional analgesia.

Patient monitoring

Dental procedures may now be initiated and carried out in an efficient yet unhurried manner. Throughout the procedure the patient will remain almost motionless. If undisturbed, he will generally have his eyes closed and may appear to be sleeping. On verbal command however, he will open his eyes and respond appropriately. All protective reflexes being active, the patient will occasionally be observed to cough, clear his throat, take a deep breath (the sigh is a normal respiratory system reflex), or adjust his position in the dental chair.

If rendered amnesic while regional analgesia is secured, a patient may express wonderment over the fact that a solution injected into his arm can anesthetize the proper area of the mouth. Most patients will be amazed to learn that multiple injections had been administered in the oral cavity.

Because consciousness is maintained throughout the conscious-sedative procedure, while protective reflexes remain intact and active, continual monitoring of vital signs is not necessary. This is not to say that patient *observation* may be omitted. The patient should be observed for his state of consciousness throughout the case. This may be done in an unobtrusive manner as dentistry progresses. Routine directions pertaining to opening or closing the mouth, turning the head, etc. will usually suffice in determining the patient's ability to appropriately respond to command.

If the operator should desire to monitor the pulse occasionally, this may easily and inconspicuously be accomplished by palpating the carotid artery in the neck (Fig. 10-2 *A*), the superficial temporal artery anterior to the tragus of the ear (Fig. 10-2, *B*), or the facial artery in the cheek (Fig. 10-2, *C*).

The blood pressure cuff is allowed to remain in place throughout the case, allowing an occasional check of the blood pressure if desired. In the event of an untoward reaction, also, the cuff is readily available and need not be applied "after the fact."

Completion of case and patient dismissal

After all dental procedures have been completed, the dental chair should slowly be adjusted from the reclining to a more upright position. After the patient has remained in this position for a brief period of time, the pulse rate and blood pressure are once again taken and recorded on his record. Should the patient experience dizziness or lightheadedness during positional change, he must be returned to the semireclining position. Usually, this is not the case.

The intravenous infusion is discontinued and the blood pressure cuff is removed. Next, the arm of the dental chair is removed or repositioned so that the patient may turn and sit for a time with feet on the floor. If no dizziness develops, he is then assisted to the standing position. Patients must not be simultaneously permitted to stand and walk from the chair. Should dizziness develop under these circumstances, a patient may stumble some distance from the dental chair. By allowing the patient to sit and then stand beside the chair, he may quickly be reseated if necessary.

The patient is then escorted from the operatory to the reception area, where he is discharged to the custody of a responsible adult. The escort should be made aware of the fact that the patient may have minimal residual drug effects and should be carefully assisted up or down stairs, while walking, and the like.

Any information the dentist wishes to tell the patient should be presented to him in writing also. Even though a very minimal drug effect is present on dismissal, the patient's attention or memory on occasion may be impaired to the point that instructions are confused or forgotten.

After the patient's dismissal a discharge note, relating the patient's condition at the time and the name of the person escorting the patient from the office, should be entered in the patient's record. Needless to say, no patient should be discharged unless his vital signs are stable and within normal limits and his sensorium is clear enough to permit ambulation without risk of harm. If necessary, the patient may be detained in the operatory or escorted to a recovery area where he may remain until his condition is satisfactory for dismissal.

The discharge note need not be unduly wordy or time-consuming; for medicolegal purposes one should be placed on the patient's record following each visit, even those in which conscious-sedation was not employed.

PEDIATRIC SEDATION

Some situations call for special consideration if the patient is to undergo dental treatment with the aid of conscious-sedation. Of note are those cases involving children. As has been mentioned, young age, per se, is not a contraindication to the intravenous administration of drugs. Indeed, this route is quite favorable for use with many apprehensive children. Owing to its accuracy of dosage, rapid onset, and predictable effect, it is the route of choice when feasible.

This does not imply that all apprehensive children are satisfactory candidates for intravenous conscious-sedation. Some children who are below the age of reason or those who, because of mental handicaps, cannot be reasoned with may very well be candidates for unconscious techniques. Nevertheless, a great many children considered to be unmanageable may satisfactorily undergo conscious-sedation administration by a combination of routes.

In accordance with the patient's age, weight, and emotional status, one may administer drugs via the oral route or the intramuscular route, which will calm sufficiently to allow an intravenous infusion to be started. The patient may then be "titrated" to the conscious-sedative state desired.

An alternative to this method may be to permit the patient to inhale nitrous oxide and oxygen until sufficient cooperation is gained to allow venipuncture to be undertaken. One may then either discontinue the inhalation route and "switch" to intravenous methods or continue the inhalation method and employ smaller drug doses administered intravenously.

In any event, the objects of conscious-sedation must be adhered to regardless of the combination of routes employed. One must always remember that differences in onset, effects, and duration are to be expected when various routes are combined and alter the technique accordingly.

For convenience in determining drug doses in children the following information is presented:

Clark's rule:

$$\frac{\text{Weight of child in pounds}}{150} \times \text{Adult dose}$$

Young's rule:

$$\frac{\text{Age of child in years}}{\text{Age} + 12} \times \text{Adult dose}$$

SUMMARY

The basic principles of intravenous conscious-sedation procedures have been presented. An attempt was made to integrate the concepts of conscious-sedation into an organized and logical sequence of events that will give favorable results in the vast majority of cases. This was done while allowing latitude concerning drug selection, doses, effects, and duration—to permit individualism and flexibility of the conscious-sedative technique.

Chapter 11

MANAGEMENT OF MEDICAL EMERGENCIES

Although emergencies in the dental office do not appear with great frequency, their occurrence is by no means rare. By definition an emergency situation may be said to be any unforeseen combination of circumstances requiring immediate attention. It should be stressed that not all emergencies are necessarily life endangering, but since an element of doubt may exist as to the final outcome, some immediate treatment is indicated. Whenever there is any deviation from the normally expected pattern, regardless of how slight, one must assume that an emergency situation is occurring. A seemingly minor complication may become a serious emergency if neglected or improperly treated.

Complications may be classified as primary or secondary, mild or severe, transient or permanent. Thus an emergency may be of a primary, mild, and transient nature or perhaps be secondary, severe, and transient. Fortunately, the vast majority of complications occurring in the dental office are either primary, mild, and transient or secondary, mild, and transient.

A *primary* complication is one that occurs and manifests itself at the time of treatment. A *secondary* complication is one that is manifested later, even though it may have been caused during initial treatment.

A *mild* complication is one that exhibits a slight deviation from the normally expected pattern and reverses itself without any specific treatment other than removing its cause. A *severe* complication manifests itself by a pronounced deviation from the normally expected pattern and requires a definite plan of therapy to reverse it.

A *transient* complication is one that may be severe at the time of occurrence but leaves no residual effect. A *permanent* complication will, of course, leave a residual effect, even though it may be mild.

The management of emergency situations may be divided into three distinct categories: (1) prevention, (2) recognition, and (3) treatment. It must be realized that each category represents an important phase of emergency management and must be thoroughly understood and appreciated if the life and welfare of the patient are to be safeguarded at all times.

PREVENTION

Without a doubt the most important phase in the management of dental office emergencies is prevention. At first glance this may appear to be a facetious statement. However, such is not the case. All too often, emergency situations are allowed to arise when their prevention could have been implemented rather easily. By taking simple precautions and devoting a minimum amount of time to the prevention of emergencies the practitioner may spare himself, in a great many instances, the necessity for rendering emergency treatment.

Several important measures may be included in dental practice that aid in the prevention of office emergency situations. Primary among these is the performance of an adequate pretreatment medical history and physical evaluation. This evaluation will alert the dentist to any physical or psychological states that may predispose the individual to the occurrence of emergency situations. Through proper evaluation the practitioner will be able to determine the presence of various conditions that alter the patient's ability to tolerate the physical and emotional stresses placed on him by dental treatment.

Today many patients who lead relatively normal, productive lives are able to do so only with pharmacotherapeutic assistance. Their pathological conditions are delicately balanced by a combination of drug therapy and moderation of physical activities. Only by understanding the pathological condition that the patient presents, by being knowledgeable concerning the pharmacology of therapeutic agents employed, and by realizing the degree of stress that will be satisfactorily tolerated can the dentist hope to prevent an emergency from developing. Determining the patient's overall ability to safely and satisfactorily undergo dental treatment must be based on a knowledge and understanding of the entire organism.

One must also realize that the system or systems in which frailties exist is the one most prone to be involved in an emergency situation. The more detailed the pretreatment evaluation, the more valuable it will be in uncovering those weaknesses, be they physical or psychological, that are most likely to be manifested during dental treatment. Realizing which weaknesses exist should offer a practitioner a good clue as to what type of emergency is most likely to develop, which system will most probably be involved, and what specific measures may be taken to prevent that specific emergency. As an example, consider the patient presenting with a history of asthma. The possibility of his experiencing an asthmatic attack while undergoing dental treatment is 100% greater than that of the nonasthmatic individual. Exposure to irritating vapors, administration of certain drugs, or a psychologically upsetting episode is likely to trigger an asthmatic attack. Prevention of this emergency might be secured by determining those types of agents to which the individual is particularly sensitive and refraining from their use. The use of conscious-sedation during dental treatment, to allay fear and apprehension, would almost preclude entirely the possibility of an asthmatic attack being initiated by psychological or emotional stress. By comparison, in the nonasthmatic individual, the likelihood of an asthmatic attack being provoked during dental treatment is nonexistent. This individual does not possess the abnormal reactive pulmonary system required to elicit asthmatic responses.

From this example one may easily appreciate the value of a thorough pretreatment evaluation in the prevention of emergencies. Analogous situations exist with almost every system in which some degree of impairment to normal function exists. It is the dentist's obligation to determine, through proper examination, the system or systems that are impaired as well as their degree of impairment. If one is to sufficiently prepare himself to prevent emergencies from developing, the history must thoroughly evaluate each major system. Questions as general as "Have you ever been told you had heart trouble?" should be avoided. Receiving a negative reply to such a query would undoubtedly give the dentist a false sense of security, since in many cases the patient may be unaware of pathological states that exist. Under such circumstances, the dentist may be the first member of the health team to detect or suspect the problem.

In other instances the patient may present with a pathological condition that, because of the regular use of therapeutic agents, goes relatively unnoticed. A generalized question to the patient may fail to uncover the presence of a potentially dangerous situation. Another measure that may be undertaken to aid in the prevention of emergencies is a proper evaluation of a patient's psychological condition. This evaluation should complement an assessment of the physical condition, for many patients present with significant impairment in both realms.

It has been stated that the vast majority of dental office emergencies are induced by psychological factors. In patients who are of sound physical condition, the untoward reaction may manifest itself as a bout of syncope. However, when the physical condition is less than optimal, psychological factors will frequently precipitate an untoward reaction that involves an already compromised system. Thus attacks of asthma, angina pectoris, epilepsy, or the like may be initiated by emotionally trying or upsetting experiences.

The role of conscious-sedation in the prevention of emergencies now becomes quite evident. Those individuals whose physical conditions are impaired are the ones who are most likely to exhibit untoward reactions, since they are least able to tolerate physically or emotionally stressful situations. In addition, these are the same patients in whom the reaction is most likely to be of a severe nature. The ability of conscious-sedation coupled with adequate regional analgesia to decrease the physical stresses of dental appointments becomes invaluable in prevention of untoward reactions in medically compromised patients.

As stated previously, psychological factors account for the initiation of the vast majority of dental office emergencies. Once again the role of conscious-sedation is to be emphasized. By alleviating fear and apprehension and reducing or eliminating psychological factors through the use of conscious-sedative techniques the prevention of virtually all office emergency situations is assured.

In summary, one may state that prevention is the best means of managing emergency situations. Prevention can best be accomplished by (1) performing an adequate pretreatment medical history and physical examination, (2) evaluating and understanding both the physical and the psychological condition of the patient, and (3) employing conscious-sedation in those patients having physical and/or psychological impairment, in order to reduce stress and anxiety.

RECOGNITION

Recognition is the second phase in the management of medical emergencies. It consists of realizing that a deviation from the normally expected pattern is occurring. Simple though this may sound, many serious emergencies are allowed to occur because the operator does not recognize minor deviations quickly. As a result the situation is inadvertently allowed to deteriorate until more obvious and severe complications are noticed. If management of emergencies is to be successfully accomplished, they must be recognized and treated as early in their course as possible. This may best be accomplished by being thoroughly familiar with the patient's preoperative condition, including the values for his "normal" vital signs. This knowledge will give the practitioner baseline values from which to identify the presence and degree of deviation that may be occurring. Without having such baseline values from which to operate, the dentist is in many instances unable to recognize the presence or seriousness of an emergency.

Since variances exist among individuals, it is difficult if not impossible to state that any one patient is "normal." What may be normal for one person is abnormal for another. Consequently, one must consider a range of values for any given parameter, within which a patient usually functions. The healthy patient with impairment to no organ or system may satisfactorily tolerate a great degree of deviation outside his "normal limits" for a brief period of time without suffering serious sequelae. On the other hand, the individual having one or more systems compromised by pathological states may not tolerate well even mild deviations in physiological function. The practitioner, therefore, must not only determine the range of normal limits within which each patient usually functions; he must also determine the patient's ability to tolerate deviations outside that range.

As an example, one may consider the importance of blood pressure values during an episode of syncope. Assume that during an episode the systolic blood pressure is recorded at 80 mm. Hg. Without a preoperative baseline value one may be unable to determine whether or not this blood pressure presents an emergency situation. Without knowing the range of normal for his patient, the practitioner may be at a loss in deciding whether or not the patient is experiencing a significant hypotensive episode.

If, however, pretreatment examination revealed the fact that the patient was in good health and this systolic blood pressure was usually around 90 mm. Hg, one may conclude that a very mild and insignificant degree of hypotension is present. Simple measures may be all that are required to correct the problem and in all probability the emergency will be transient, leaving no residual effects. On the other hand a pretreatment systolic blood pressure of 180 mm. Hg would indicate the presence of a rather severe hypotensive episode that, if not quickly and properly rectified, is almost certain to result in a permanent complication, which may be of a primary and/or a secondary nature.

When employing conscious-sedation one must be thoroughly familiar with the pharmacology of agents being administered. One must realize that although the incidence of adverse reactions to drugs being administered is extremely low, all are capable of producing untoward reactions. In most instances the reaction produced will be directly attributable to the agent and is usually the result of too great a dose and/or a too rapid rate of administration. Only by understanding the pharmacology of the agent and by being able to recognize the usual response to that agent is one able to distinguish usual from unusual responses.

In some individuals atropine administration will result in a red, blotchy appearance of the skin of the face, neck, and shoulder area. The uninformed practitioner may mistakenly interpret this reaction as being an allergic response. Knowledge of appropriate pharmacology would indicate that this response is frequently apparent, due to the ability of atropine to dilate the microcirculation of the blush area. In this example, therefore, the presence of a "rash" is unexpected only because of a lack of adequate information. The knowledgeable clinician would not have considered an untoward reaction or an emergency situation to be present.

Although prevention is the best means of managing emergency situations, the importance of *early* recognition is to be stressed. Factors that will enable the practitioner to recognize the presence and severity of an emergency include the following: (1) use of the pretreatment medical history and physical examination to establish "normal, baseline" parameters; (2) appreciation of the "range of normal limits," within which the patient must function; (3) realization of the patient's ability to tolerate deviations outside his "normal limits"; (4) early identification of a set of circumstances as an emergency situation.

TREATMENT

The third phase of emergency management involves the initiation of any measures that are required for correcting physiological deviations that may be detrimental to the life or welfare of the patient. The treatment phase may be further divided into two categories: management of emergencies *without* the use of drugs and management of emergencies *with* the use of drugs.

Management of emergencies without the use of drugs

There is no doubt within my mind that the vast majority of emergencies occurring within the dental office can be satisfactorily managed *without* the use of drugs. Fifteen years of experience coupled with the opportunity to manage or supervise the management of thousands of dental cases with and without the use of conscious-sedation attest to this statement.

This does not mean that emergency management that requires the use of drugs may be ignored. To the contrary. It means that one must constantly ready himself, through appropriate learning procedures, to cope with those emergencies that require definitive drug therapy. Because of their infrequent occurrence one is likely to be "out of practice" when such a situation arises if rigorous attention to the necessary knowledge and skills is allowed to wane.

In correctly managing emergency situations that do not require the use of drugs, attention must be paid to proper methodology, applied in proper sequence. The sequence is simple to remember, since the steps are applied in alphabetical order. All office personnel should be thoroughly familiar with and trained in this aspect of emergency management.

A = *Airway*. Appropriate steps must be taken to ensure the patency of the airway, thus allowing the free passage of air into and out of the lungs.

B = *Breathing*. The patient should be observed for the presence of adequate breathing. This means that inspiratory and expiratory efforts must be accompanied by adequate pulmonary ventilation. Assisted or controlled ventilation may be necessary.

C = *Circulation*. The status of the patient's circulatory system must be evaluated and supported as required.

D = *Definitive* measures are instituted.

Each aspect of the emergency management will now be discussed in detail.

Airway

Most serious emergencies that are likely to occur in the dental office and that can be managed without the use of drugs will, in almost every instance, involve an unconscious patient.

When he is in this state, regardless of its cause, the patient will invariably assume a position in which the muscles of the neck relax and allow the head to flex. The tongue literally falls posteriorly against the posterior pharyngeal wall, resulting in obstruction of the airway. (See Fig. 11-1, *A*.) This type of obstruction is the most common cause of asphyxia in the unconscious patient.

Some patients may have a partial airway obstruction produced by the same mechanism. If it is allowed to continue, the obstruction may result in the more gradual production of hypoxia.

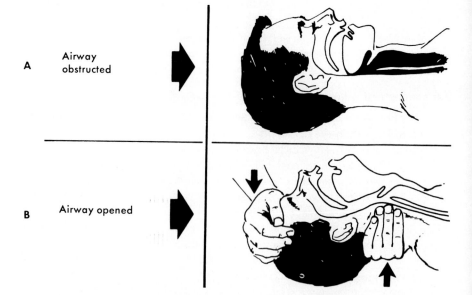

Airway
obstructed

A

Airway opened

B

Fig. 11-1. A, Obstruction of the airway by soft tissue in the unconscious patient.
B, Maximum backward tilt of the head provides a patent airway. (Courtesy Statham
Instruments, Inc.)

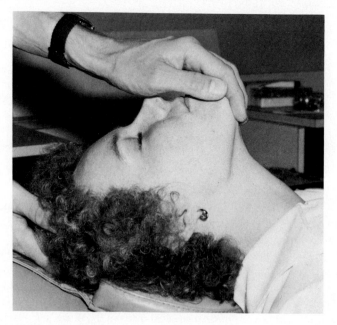

Fig. 11-2. Placing one hand under the chin and the other on the forehead provides
maximum head extension.

In the patient in need of airway assistance the following steps should be carried out in rapid sequence:

1. One hand should be placed under the neck or under the chin and the other on the forehead.
2. Maximum backward tilt (neck extension) of the head should be accomplished. *This is the single most important step in managing the unconscious patient.* It moves the mandible forward and stretches the anterior neck structures and lifts the base of the tongue from the posterior pharyngeal wall. (See Figs. 11-1, *B*, and 11-2.) Maximum neck extension provides an open air passage in 80% of unconscious subjects.
3. Forward displacement (protrusion) of the mandible may aid in the maintenance of a patent airway. The patient's chin may be lifted by using one hand with a finger or the thumb in the subject's mouth (Fig. 11-3), or the mandible may be protruded by applying pressure with both hands at angles of the mandible. The optimal airway is provided by a combination of maximum backward tilt of the head coupled with protrusion of the mandible and separation of the teeth and lips (Fig. 11-4).
4. Clearing the pharynx of any foreign matter that may be present must

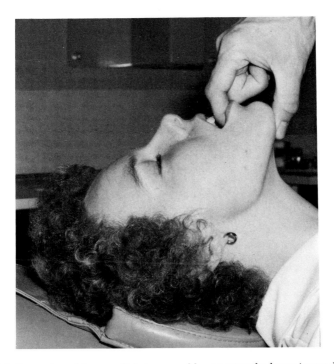

Fig. 11-3. Protrusion of the mandible is secured by grasping the lower jaw and pulling it forward.

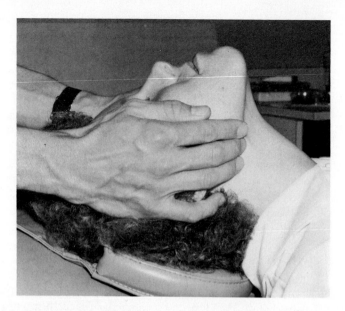

Fig. 11-4. Optimal airway provided by a combination of maximum backward tilt of the head, coupled with protrusion of the mandible by forward pressure at angles.

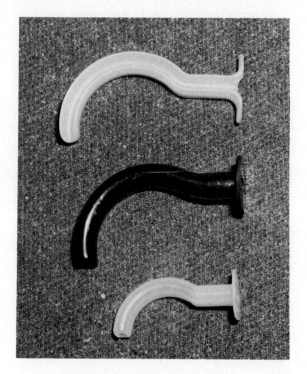

Fig. 11-5. Oropharyngeal airways.

accompany the maneuvers already described. In the dental office this can be easily accomplished with the aid of a suction apparatus.

5. If maintenance of the airway appears to be difficult, an oropharyngeal airway (Fig. 11-5) may be inserted (Fig. 11-6). These airways are used to hold the base of the tongue forward and prevent obstruction caused by the lips and teeth. Even with the oropharyngeal airway in place, the neck must be maximally extended.

In the event that airway obstruction is being caused by a foreign body that has been inhaled, in all probability the object will be lodged at the glottal opening. This opening, which is located between the vocal cords, is the narrowest opening in the upper airway of the adult. All efforts previously described will be of no avail in this situation. The patient will usually be attempting to make violent but unsuccessful respiratory movements. He will be stricken with fear, and death is imminent if the obstruction is not relieved quickly.

Under circumstances of this dire emergency one must perform a *cricothyroidotomy* to enable the free passage of air. A cricothyroidotomy trochar (Fig. 11-7) or an emergency tracheal catheter (Fig. 11-8) is inserted into the airway in the midline through the cricothyroid membrane, a structure that lies between the thyroid and cricoid cartilages. When using the emergency tracheal catheter, the head is extended and the appropriate struc-

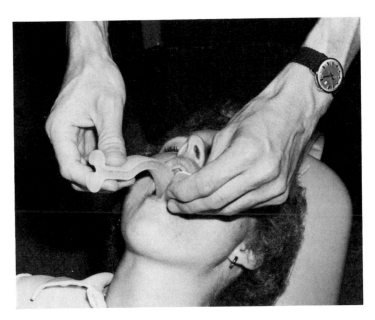

Fig. 11-6. Tongue blade being used to assist insertion of oropharyngeal airway.

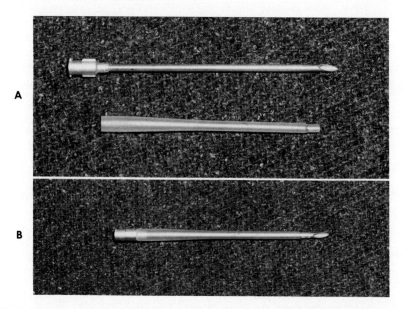

Fig. 11-7. Emergency cricothyroidotomy needle. A 12-gauge needle with 10-gauge sheath that remains in place after needle within it is removed following cricothyroidotomy.

tures identified. The 12-gauge needle with the 10-gauge catheter over it is introduced into the airway. Once positioned, the needle is withdrawn, leaving the catheter in place to provide an emergency airway below the occluded glottal opening. Hospitalization for removal of the foreign body and definitive care must follow.

Breathing

After performing the steps required to establish a patent airway, the operator must direct his attention to the patient's breathing. Very often, establishing a patent airway is all that is necessary to treat the emergency. However, one must be certain that respiratory effects are present and adequate.

Most presently recommended methods of artificial ventilation depend on intermittent inflation of the lungs with positive pressure applied to the airway. Ideally, airway pressure should return to atmospheric level between positive pressure inflations. The forces opposing inflation that must be overcome are the elastic resistance of the lungs and thorax and airway resistance. Shallow, inadequate respiration may be augmented with positive pressure inflations, whereas apnea must be treated with controlled ventilation. Ventilation may be assisted or controlled using exhaled air, atmospheric air, or oxygen.

The properly equipped dental office should contain a mechanical device, such as the Ambu Resuscitator (Fig. 11-9) or the Puritan Manual Resuscitator

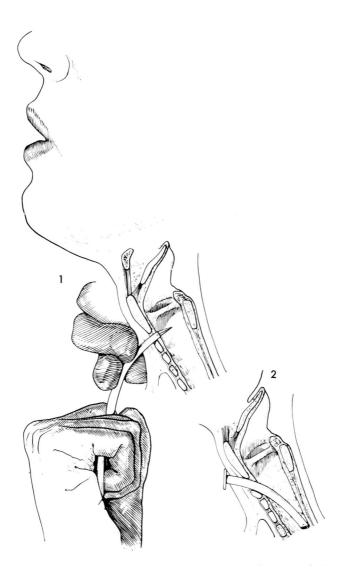

Fig. 11-8. Cricothyroidotomy for emergency tracheostomy. *1,* Insertion of cricothyroid-otomy trocar. *2,* Cricothyroidotomy tube in place. (From Bennett, C. R.: Monheim's general anesthesia in dental practice, ed. 4, St. Louis, 1974, The C. V. Mosby Co.)

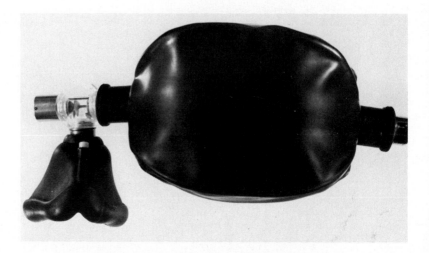

Fig. 11-9. Ambu Resuscitator.

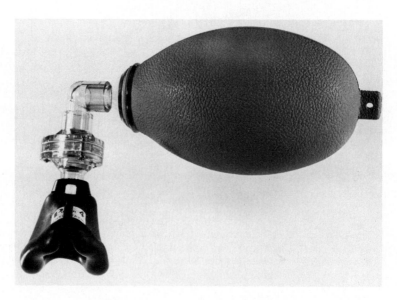

Fig. 11-10. Puritan Manual Resuscitator.

(Fig. 11-10), for application of artificial ventilation. Such devices are, essentially, air pumps that allow the operator to artificially ventilate the subject's lungs with atmospheric air. Because of the arrangement of various valves, air contained in the breathing bag will be forced through the mask and into the patient's lungs when the bag is squeezed. When the patient exhales through the mask, the air is directed into the atmosphere by the valve arrangement. The bag refills with atmospheric air when manual pressure is released. The patient, therefore, can neither deplete the oxygen nor accumulate carbon dioxide in the breathing bag. These manual ventilators are also equipped with adapters that can be connected to an oxygen source, permitting artificial ventilation with an oxygen-enriched mixture if desired. An analgesia machine may also be used as a means of providing artificial ventilation. When used with either a full face mask or a nasal inhaler, the analgesia machine is capable of delivering positive pressure lung inflations with 100% oxygen.

In the absence of a suitable device for artificially inflating the lungs, exhaled air from the operator may be breathed into the patient to supply adequate ventilation.

The following steps are followed when employing assisted or controlled ventilation:

1. The neck is extended to its fullest, and patency of the airway is established as described under the discussion on airway.

2. When using mouth-to-mouth ventilation, the operator takes a deep breath, seals his mouth around the patient's mouth (which falls open with neck extension), and exhales forcefully into the patient (Fig. 11-11). When blowing into the patient's mouth, the operator must pinch the subject's nostrils closed to prevent air leakage.

3. The operator observes the subject's chest during inflation. After the chest expands to its fullest, the patient is allowed to exhale passively while the operator takes another deep breath in preparation for the next inflation.

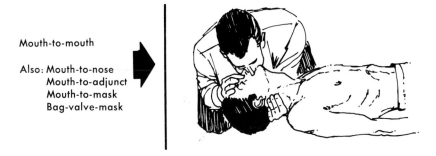

Mouth-to-mouth

Also: Mouth-to-nose
　　　Mouth-to-adjunct
　　　Mouth-to-mask
　　　Bag-valve-mask

Fig. 11-11. Mouth-to-mouth ventilation. Other types of emergency ventilation also listed. (Courtesy Statham Instruments, Inc.)

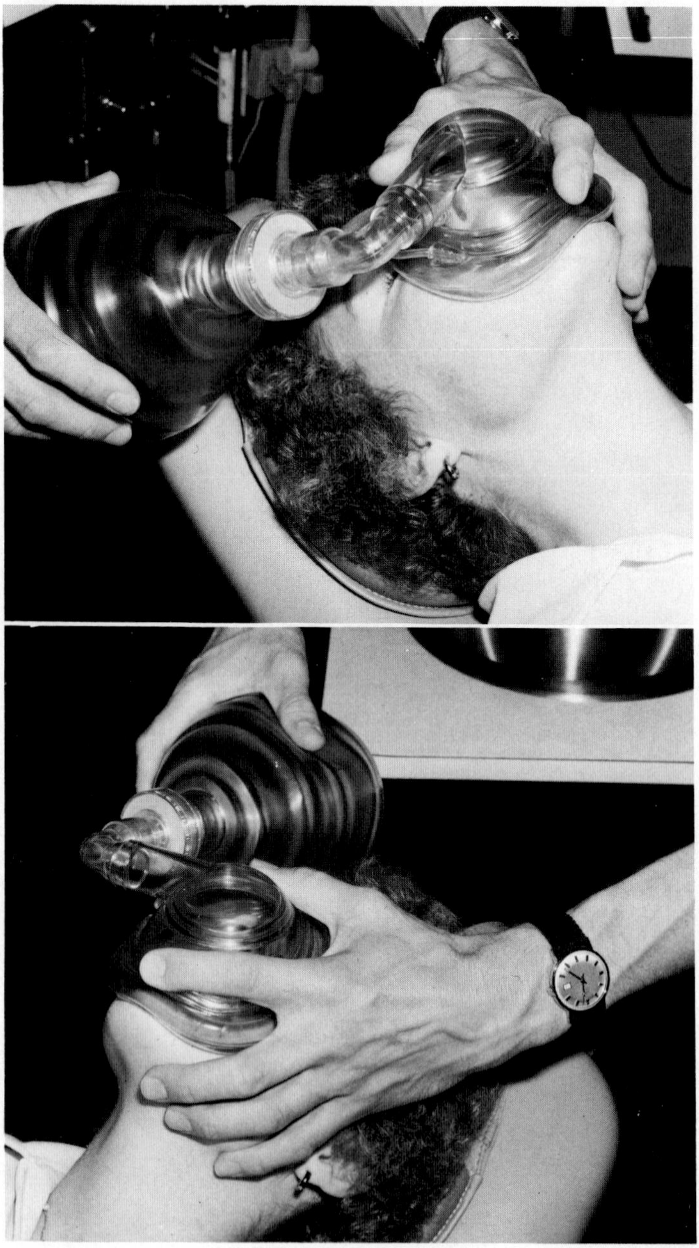

Fig. 11-12. Left hand clamps mask to face and extends head while right hand squeezes bag to inflate lungs.

4. If assisted ventilation is being employed, the operator exhales into the subject during every third or fourth spontaneous inhalation. Controlled ventilation would be applied once every 5 seconds.
5. When a manual ventilator is used to provide the inspiratory effort, the mask is applied to the subject's face with one hand. The neck is extended to maintain the airway in a patent state, and the hand is used to clamp the mask tightly to the patient's face (Fig. 11-12). With the operator's free hand the bag is squeezed until the patient's chest rises; then the bag is rapidly released to permit exhalation. When a nasal mask at-

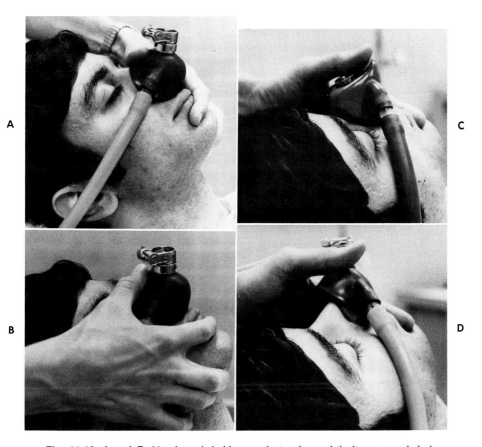

A

B

C

D

Fig. 11-13. A and **B,** Nasal mask held securely in place while lips are sealed shut. Maximum neck extension provides a patent airway. **C,** Thumb pressure holds exhalation valve shut while providing a secure mask fit. **D,** During exhalation, mask is lightly lifted from the face to allow patient to exhale into atmosphere.

tached to an analgesia machine is employed for artificial ventilation, the mask must be held firmly in place over the nose while the lips are sealed shut as well (Fig. 11-13, *A* and *B*). This step prevents air from leaking from the mouth during positive pressure lung inflations. During artificial ventilation the exhalation valve and the rebreathing port must also be adjusted to the closed position. Maximum neck extension is coupled with this maneuver to provide a patent airway. On those masks not having an adjustable exhalation valve, the left thumb must hold the valve shut as well as aid in securing the mask in position (Fig. 11-13, *C*). To prevent rebreathing during exhalation the mask must be lightly lifted from the patient's face (Fig. 11-13, *D*) or thumb pressure be released from the exhalation valve when the patient exhales. Since rebreathing does not occur, high flow rates (6 to 10 liters per minute) of 100% oxygen must be used to rapidly fill the breathing bag with sufficient oxygen for controlled ventilation.

To this point the management of emergencies without the use of drugs has dealt exclusively with managing problems associated with respiration, since in most instances it is the respiratory apparatus that is the first to suffer in emergency situations. Careful attention to maintenance of the airway coupled with ensuring adequate ventilation will resolve the emergency in most cases. These steps prevent the occurrence of hypoxia, which if allowed to persist is certain to result in deterioration of the circulatory system.

Although support of the circulatory system will be discussed, it is imperative that one appreciate the *extreme importance* of quickly and efficiently performing the steps just described *first*.

Circulation

In most instances in which circulatory support is required for maintaining blood pressure within normal limits, proper patient positioning coupled with respiratory system assistance is all that is required. Hypotension encountered

Check pulse

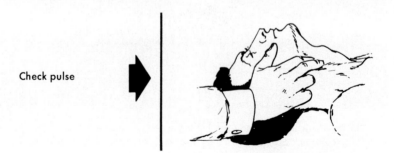

Fig. 11-14. Status of circulatory system is assessed by palpating the carotid pulse.

in the dental office is invariably caused by a maldistribution of blood volume coupled with dilation of the microcirculation. This combination may be psychologically (syncope) or pharmacologically induced. The net effect is a decrease in venous return accompanied by a fall in cardiac output, blood pressure, cerebral perfusion, and oxygenation. Should this chain of events occur in a patient seated upright or standing, consciousness will be rapidly lost and collapse of the patient is imminent.

Proper treatment of this condition involves taking measures to increase venous return to the heart, thereby encouraging normal circulatory reflexes to correct the problem.

Proper chair position is usually all that is required to take advantage of gravitational forces to increase venous return. Elevation of the legs can increase venous return by 500 to 700 ml. per leg, while elevation of the upper extremities may add 200 to 300 ml. per arm. Adjusting the dental chair to such a position that both the thorax and legs are slightly elevated (Fig. 11-15) provides an "autotransfusion" by dumping venous blood pooled in the peripheral circulation into the great vessels returning to the heart.

In my experience I have never seen patients already seated in this position lose consciousness under ordinary dental office circumstances. However, they may experience syncope, manifested by lightheadedness, pallor, perspiration, and the like. If the patient in this position is instructed to breath deeply, ve-.

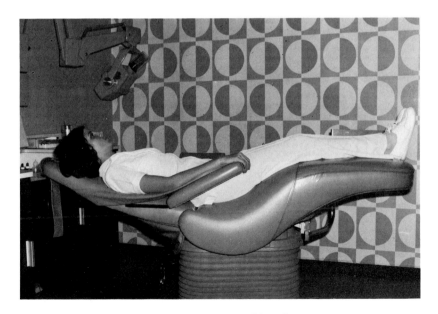

Fig. 11-15. Reclining chair position used for aiding venous return.

nous return is further increased by activating the thoracic pump mechanism—increasing the negative intrathoracic pressure during inspiration—thereby further aiding venous return. The position described, not unlike the one assumed when reclining in a hammock, also makes spontaneous, assisted, or controlled ventilation easier by removing the weight of the abdominal viscera from the inferior surface of the diaphragm, a situation that occurs when the patient is placed in the conventional Trendelenburg position in which the entire body is inclined head down at about 15 degrees.

Most frequently this mechanical aid to circulation is all that is required to correct the situation. Fluids, vasoconstrictors, and anticholinergic drugs may be administered if required and will be discussed later.

In the event the patient is found to be pulseless on palpation of the carotid pulse, one must institute external cardiac compression.

Rationale. The heart occupies most of the space between the sternum and the vertebral column. Artificial circulation is produced by squeezing the heart between these two structures as sternal compression is applied. Blood is thereby forced out of the left ventricle into the body. When the pressure is released, the elasticity of the chest wall causes the thorax to expand and the heart refills with blood.

The procedures to be followed when performing external cardiac compression (Fig. 11-16) are discussed here:

1. The operator positions himself to either side of the patient.
2. To be effective and prevent damage during compression, pressure must be applied at exactly the center of the lower half of the sternum. The heel of one hand is placed over the pressure point and the heel of the other hand is placed on top of the first.
3. The sternum is pushed downward about 1½ to 2 inches in adults, then released rapidly. Pressure is applied every second or slightly faster. Rates slower than 60 per minute do not provide sufficient blood flow. In adults, the pressure is applied by using the entire weight of the body, delivered as a blow from the shoulders. The patient must be positioned on a firm surface for external cardiac compression to be effective. Most modern dental chairs are acceptable.

The hands are not removed from the sternum between compressions. Compression must be forceful enough to produce good carotid or femoral artery pulses. Rhythmic compression should not be interrupted except for a few seconds, since the amount of circulation produced is only 20% to 40% of normal.

External cardiac compression alone does not produce ventilation of the lungs and therefore must be combined with intermittent positive pressure ventilation. Recommended rates and rations of ventilation and sternal compression aim at optimal function as well as technical feasibility.

The ratio for one operator is two lung inflations followed by fifteen sternal

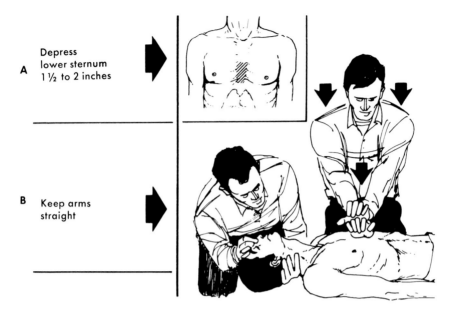

A

Depress
lower sternum
1 ½ to 2 inches

B

Keep arms
straight

Fig. 11-16. A, Pressure point for application of external cardiac compression. Pressure must be applied exactly over the center of the lower half of the sternum. **B,** Operator positioned for application of external cardiac compression. (Courtesy Statham Instruments, Inc.)

compressions at 2-second intervals. If there are two operators, one of them compresses the sternum at 1-second intervals without interruption. The ventilating operator interposes one deep lung inflation after every fifth sternal compression.

Every 2 minutes the procedure should be interrupted to check for return of spontaneous pulse. Cardiopulmonary resuscitation should be continued until spontaneous pulse returns. Artificial ventilation without compression should continue until spontaneous breathing returns. Oxygen, perhaps with positive pressure assistance, should be administered until the patient regains consciousness.

If the victim can be resuscitated and if the resuscitative efforts are effective, the pupils will usually constrict; the victim's color will improve. Constriction of the pupils is the most encouraging sign that adequate circulation of oxygenated blood is being maintained. Movement by the victim obviously indicates that there are adequate circulation and viability of the brain.

As soon as all steps described above have been established and are continuing without interruption, efforts should be made to start definitive measures.

Definitive measures (drugs are included)

When cardiopulmonary resuscitation is still required after 5 minutes, the following steps should be taken:

1. An intravenous infusion should be started.
2. Administer 0.5 to 1 mg. of epinephrine intravenously. This dose may be repeated every 5 to 10 minutes. Epinephrine will be useful in the presence of either asystole or fibrillation. It aids in maintaining blood pressure and improving myocardial tone.
3. Administer 50 ml. doses of sodium bicarbonate intravenously every 10 minutes. This acts to combat acidosis, which always occurs during cardiopulmonary resuscitation.
4. Summon assistance and transport victim to hospital as soon as possible. Every effort should be made not to interrupt artificial ventilation and artificial circulation. If adequate spontaneous respiration and pulse return, there is no need to persist with emergency techniques. However, if they again disapper reinstitute emergency measures.

Although the previous discussion of emergency management includes heroic measures that may be required, need for them is the exception rather than the rule. Not infrequently, however the dentist may be called on to institute the rather simple but extremely important emergency measures discussed in earlier portions of the chapter.

The early, simple measures taken to treat medical emergencies can be likened to helping a child climb a tree. If the child is unable to reach the lowest limb, the prospects for him climbing the tree are rather poor. However, if one offers a boost, in all probability the child will climb the tree easily. The mechanical maneuvers described are analogous to boosting a faltering physiology. If one can offer a little assistance at the outset of the emergency, in all probability the patient's reflexes will be boosted to the point where normal function resumes and the emergency then corrects itself.

Careful attention to prevention and recognition of emergencies coupled with prompt and efficient treatment without the use of drugs will obviate the need for elaborate measures in most instances.

Management of emergencies that may require the use of drugs

The number of emergencies occuring in the dental office that require the use of drugs in their management is extremely low. Nevertheless, the dentist must be familiar with them so that he may be able to take appropriate measures to safeguard the welfare of the patient. In every instance, those appropriate mechanical methods already described should be employed initially in an attempt to correct the situation. In many instances both mechanical and pharmacological methods must be utilized.

Conditions most likely to produce emergency situations in the dental office, which require the use of drugs, involve the following:

I. Respiratory system
   A. Allergy
   B. Asthma
II. Cardiovascular system
   A. Hypotension
   B. Bradycardia
   C. Syncope
   D. Arteriolosclerotic heart disease
      1. Angina pectoris
      2. Coronary artery occlusion
III. Nervous system
   A. Stimulation
      1. Epilepsy
      2. Drug-induced reaction
   B. Depression
   C. Cerebral vascular accidents
IV. Endocrine system
   A. Diabetes mellitus
      1. Insulin shock
      2. Diabetic coma
   B. Adrenal insufficiency

Respiratory system emergencies

When a respiratory emergency occurs it will usually result from a preexisting condition plus an exaggerating factor or circumstance, such as emotion or introduction of an allergen. The first concern must be to determine whether respiratory exchange is adequate and take the appropriate mechanical steps outlined before.

Allergy. Allergy may be defined as a specific hypersensitivity to a specific agent or to one of similar chemical derivation, based on a true antigen-antibody reaction. This type of emergency is comparatively uncommon; it has been estimated that less than 1% of all reactions occurring when regional analgesia is employed are allergic in origin.

An allergy may be acquired or familial and embraces most forms of specific hypersensitivity, including anaphylactoid shock. The skin, mucous membranes, and blood vessels are (as a rule) the shock organs; and as a result the symptoms are manifested by urticaria, wheals, edema, migraine, and in some cases respiratory distress.

The allergic response may be mild or severe. Generally, the first allergic reaction is a mild one, with succeeding responses being more severe.

Treatment for an allergic reaction is determined by the type of reaction exhibited. If the reaction is an extremely mild one, no treatment may be required. If an immediate rash, urticaria, or edema of the angioneurotic type is manifested, an antihistamine such as diphenhydramine (Benadryl) in 20 to 50 mg. doses should be administered at the time of the symptoms.

Steroid hormones such as hydrocortisone (Solu-Cortef) in 100 mg. doses administered intravenously are also beneficial, since these agents have antihistaminic properties and decrease the inflammatory reaction.

For those allergic reactions involving the tracheobronchial tree that occur in the nonasthmatic patient, the use of intravenous antihistamines and the steroid hormones should suffice. These reactions are usually more annoying than serious. Lacrimation, sneezing, and rhinorrhea that are exhibited are easily controlled with conservative drug therapy.

Asthma. It is stated that over 50% of all cases of bronchial asthma occur as the result of an allergy to external antigens. Asthma may range from mild to severe and is manifested by a wheezing type of respiration, with expiration much more affected than inspiration. An attack may be precipitated by exposure to a specific allergen, unusual excitement, emotional stress, or infection. A mild attack producing no prolonged respiratory distress should require no specific treatment. However, if the condition is more severe and breathing is a problem, some emergency treatment is indicated.

Many asthmatic patients who have frequent attacks carry an isoproterenol inhaler (Isuprel Mistometer) with them to be used in alleviating their symptoms. If such is the case, the patient should be allowed to treat the attack himself. He is much more familiar with the situation and is more capable of treating the attack than anyone else.

In the event the patient does not carry such medication, the dentist should provide an isoproterenol inhaler and allow the patient to take several deep inhalations from the nebulizer.

Alternative treatment would include the administration of intravenous aminophylline. One may place 500 mg. in a 500 ml. bottle of 5% dextrose in water and administer it carefully. This drug will quickly alleviate the respiratory distress. However, since it also dilates the microcirculation, it must be administered with caution lest it produce an undesirable hypotensive episode.

For severe asthmatic attacks that do not respond to more conservative treatment, the intramuscular administration of 0.3 to 0.5 mg. of epinephrine is indicated. Since this is an extremely potent drug, care must be taken to avoid inadvertent intravenous injection of this dose.

Cardiovascular system emergencies

Cardiovascular system emergencies usually involve those patients having a degree of cardiovascular system impairment. However, some emergency situations may arise in the healthy individual as well.

Hypotension. As described earlier, every attempt should be made to manage hypotensive episodes through the use of positional changes and adequate oxygenation. Rarely, these measures will not suffice and pharmacological assistance will be required. Under conditions of hypotension the intravenous route is almost mandatory, since absorption by other routes will be slow and unpredictable as a result of poor tissue perfusion.

Drugs that will prove to be most beneficial are phenylephrine (Neo-Synephrine) and methoxamine (Vasoxyl).

Phenylephrine may be administered intravenously via the "wash" technique. With this technique 1 ml. of phenylephrine is drawn into a 3 ml. syringe. The drug is then deposited back into its original container. The same needle and syringe are then used for venipuncture and 3 ml. of blood is drawn into the syringe. The blood and the phenylephrine that adhered to the walls of the needle and syringe after expulsion of the drug are then "washed" into the vein. A pressor effect will follow shortly.

A phenylephrine drip may also be made by placing 1 to 2 ml. of a 1:500 solution in 250 to 500 ml. of 5% dextrose in water. This may then be administered slowly with the drip rate being adjusted to produce the desired effect.

Methoxamine may also be administered intravenously in 10 to 20 mg. doses to produce a vasoconstrictor response. Through its alpha-adrenergic stimulating effect methoxamine will elevate blood pressure and produce a reflex fall in heart rate as well.

Bradycardia. Bradycardia, or slowing of the pulse rate to 50 per minute or lower, may occur with little warning. If the pulse rate is sufficient to maintain adequate cardiac output, no symptoms may be exhibited. However, if the slowed pulse is unable to maintain adequate cardiac output, hypotension, dizziness, and shortness of breath may be demonstrated. If bradycardia exists in the absence of precordial pain or other symptoms, intravenous administration of 0.2 to 0.4 mg. of atropine will correct the situation.

Syncope. Fainting, or syncope, is one of the most frequent emergencies in the dental office. This is a form of neurogenic shock and is caused by cerebral ischemia secondary to vasodilation and an increase in the vascular bed with a corresponding fall in blood pressure. When the patient is sitting upright in the dental chair, the brain is placed in a superior position and is most susceptible to the reduced blood flow.

Fainting is not always associated with loss of consciousness, since the patient may feel faint and nauseated even though he is in harmony with his surroundings. Loss of consciousness is a severe manifestation of cerebral hypoxia that is sufficient to interfere with cortical function.

The proper time to treat this complication is in its very early phases, before the patient has lost consciousness. In most instances, it is possible to detect some change in the patient's appearance, such as pallor. He may also complain of feeling strange or different. At this point one should immediately initiate the mechanical means necessary to manage the situation. Evaluation of the respiratory system must be accomplished first. Since the patient is capable of talking, one must assume that the airway is patent and spontaneous respiration is present.

The patient should quickly be positioned as described, to aid in the support of the circulatory system, and should be requested to take a few deep breaths to ensure adequate oxygenation. This simple treatment usually suffices. Soon the patient regains his normal feeling and state of consciousness. He should then be reassured and reevaluated before work is continued.

Whenever a patient loses consciousness unexpectedly in the dental chair, his pulse, respiration, and color should be checked to determine the severity of the condition. With respirations of a satisfactory rate, depth, and character, the pulse palpable with sufficient volume, the rate within reasonable limits, no arrhythmias present that were not present before, and the color satisfactory, it can be assumed that no serious accident has occurred.

If there is any marked change in respiratory pattern, accompanied by cyanosis, pallor, or ashen gray color associated with extreme tachycardia, bradycardia, or other arrhythmia not previously present, or if the pulse is weak or not palpable, one can be certain that something more severe than syncope has occurred. All necessary steps previously decribed must be instituted immediately and assistance summoned.

On occasion, however, positional change alone is inadequate to correct mild hypotension. This is usually seen in those patients having afternoon appointments who have had little to eat or drink prior to arrival at the office. These individuals may be somewhat hypoglycemic and hypovolemic as well. In addition to a relative hypovolemia caused by maldistribution of blood volume and a dilated microcirculation, their total blood volume may be deficient by 500 to 1,000 ml. Those cases refractory to correction by positional change alone may benefit by the rapid intravenous infusion of a sufficient volume of 5% dextrose in water or dextrose in lactated Ringer's solution to replace the fluid deficit.

Generally speaking, however, the management of simple syncope, the most common of all dental office emergencies, may be satisfactorily accomplished without the use of *any* medications.

Angina pectoris. Angina pectoris is characterized by the sudden onset of substernal pain, which may radiate to the left shoulder and arm and quite frequently to the left side of the neck and face. The pain is usually quite severe but may be described in referred areas as an aching type of discomfort. It is further characterized by short duration and almost immediate relief by oxygen and/or nitrites or nitroglycerin (gr. 1/150) sublingually. Patients carrying medication for such emergencies should be allowed to treat the symptoms themselves. Symptomatic relief should be obtained within a few minutes. If relief is not obtained, the possibility of coronary artery occlusion should be considered.

Coronary artery occlusion. Coronary artery occlusion may vary from mild to very severe attacks and may masquerade under various misleading signs. Substernal pain is the most common sign and symptom. In some instances the patient may experience a severe painful pressure on the chest. In milder cases coronary artery occlusion may be manifested as a "digestive crisis" or heartburn. It is not uncommon for a mild case of coronary artery occlusion to be manifested by sweating, generalized discomfort, and weakness.

In cases of coronary artery occlusion, it is not possible to depend entirely on blood pressure as a diagnostic aid, since in many cases the pressure may be within normal limits.

If the dentist thinks that the patient is in the throes of coronary artery occlusion, be it mild or severe, oxygen should be administered to help alleviate myocardial ischemia. This in itself may help to relieve the pain. The patient should be placed in a supine position with the head and thorax elevated. The relief of pain and anxiety is essential and thus morphine (8 to 15 mg.) or 50 to 100 mg. of meperidine (Demerol) should be slowly administered intravenously. Assistance should be summoned and the patient transported to a hospital for further evaluation and treatment.

Nervous system emergencies

Nervous system emergencies that are likely to be encountered may occur in the individual with a predisposition to the condition or may occur in the healthy individual as a result of drug administration.

Stimulation. Stimulation of the central nervous system may be either mild or severe and may be induced by preexisting factors such as epilepsy or may be a drug-induced phenomenon.

Epilepsy. Epilepsy occurs in about 0.5% of the population and is characterized by a loss of consciousness, involuntary muscle movements, and disturbances of the autonomic nervous system. The pretreatment evaluation should forewarn the dentist of the epileptic patient.

GRAND MAL CONVULSIONS. Grand mal seizures are characterized by excessive muscular activity, loss of consciousness, and muscle rigidity. The patient may become apneic. After an attack he may fall into an exhausted sleep or exhibit headache, vomiting, and muscle soreness. It is not uncommon for the patient to have a feeling or a warning that he is about to experience a seizure.

PETIT MAL CONVULSIONS. A petit mal convulsion is not just a small seizure but is of a different type entirely. Loss of consciousness is the predominant symptom. The eyelids, and sometimes the head, move synchronously. The seizure lasts for only a brief period (seconds), and the patient usually reacts without after-effects. He gives a history of previous attacks and the dentist is thus forewarned.

Drug-induced stimulation. Drug-induced stimulation of the central nervous system is most frequently seen after administration of a toxic dose of a local anesthetic agent. Mild stimulation if first manifested by apprehension, talkativeness, and giddiness. Mild increases in blood pressure and pulse and respiratory rates soon follow. More severe reaction is typified by a greater degree of stimulation, which may rapidly progress to generalized convulsion. Following the seizure, a period of postictal depression ensues, in which depression of the central nervous system and of the vital functions predominates.

The treatment for the convulsive type emergencies will be discussed together, since they are all very similar and require the same treatment. Important considerations are to maintain a patent airway, ensure adequate respiration, and prevent any bodily harm from occurring during the seizure.

Mild central nervous system stimulation may be controlled with the intravenous administration of ultrashort-acting barbiturates. Methohexital or thiopental may be administered in small doses until stimulation subsides.

In severe convulsive disorders the intravenous or intramuscular administration of 20 to 40 mg. of succinylcholine chloride may be required to terminate the seizure. This neuromuscular blocking agent will stop muscular seizure activity by paralyzing all voluntary muscles. Whenever this agent is employed, maintenance of the airway coupled with artificial ventilation must be applied until the drug effects are dissipated.

Depression. Depression of the central nervous system usually follows those emergencies whose primary manifestation was stimulation. In addition one may see depression of the central nervous system as a direct effect of overdose of psychosedatives, barbiturates, or narcotic analgetics.

Depression is manifested as sleepiness, lethargy, respiratory system inadequacy, and hypotension. Regardless of the cause of central nervous system depression, treatment is the same. Necessary mechanical procedures described earlier (maintain a patent airway, support respiration, and support circulation) must be instituted immediately.

As a general rule these measures will suffice without the use of drugs being necessary. If required, vasopressors may be employed. However, the use of central nervous system–stimulating drugs (analeptics) should be avoided. These agents are usually of little value, give the practitioner a false sense of security, and may on occasion produce undesirable effects.

Cerebral vascular accidents. Cerebral vascular accidents have been known to occur in the dental office. The handling of this type of emergency is primarily a case of recognition coupled with maintenance of a patent airway and adequate ventilation until definitive treatment can be rendered. These cases may be recognized from symptoms such as muscular weakness or paralysis of extremities, sudden flaccid paralysis of the side of the face, or development of slurred speech. In some cases severe unilateral headache precedes other symptoms. Treatment should consist of using those mechanical techniques described earlier and hospitalization of the patient.

Endocrine system emergencies

The endocrine system emergencies most likely to produce an office emergency are diabetes mellitus and adrenal insufficiency. Pretreatment evaluation should warn the practitioner of the presence of either condition.

Diabetes mellitus. Diabetes mellitus is a common condition affecting between 1.5% and 2% of the population. It is caused by a disorder of carbohydrate metabolism, resulting from an insulin deficiency that produces hyperglycemia and glycosuria.

Insulin shock. This emergency is brought on by a hypoglycemic state, resulting from inadequate food intake after routine insulin dosage. Signs of impending insulin shock are hunger, weakness, inability to focus the eyes, and a cold perspiration. The patient may show anger and become easily irritated or mentally confused.

At the earliest signs of the possibility of insulin shock the conscious patient should be given a few pieces of candy or a sugared drink. This will quickly correct the situation. In some instances insulin shock will appear with explosive suddenness. The patient who appeared normal one instant will be unconscious the next. In these cases, the patient should be given 0.5 to 1 mg. of glucagon hydrochloride intravenously or intramuscularly. In addition an intravenous infusion of 5% or 10% dextrose in water should be started. When the blood sugar content is elevated to suitable levels, the patient will regain consciousness as abruptly as it was lost. Under no circumstances should one attempt to administer anything by mouth to an unconscious patient. The intravenous route is preferred in such cases.

Diabetic coma. Diabetic coma occurs as a result of inadequate insulin production or intake by a severely diabetic patient. This emergency will probably never be experienced in the dental office, because of two factors. First, hyperglycemia is tolerated much better than hypoglycemia. A slight fall in blood sugar levels may produce no discernible symptoms. Second, diabetic coma does not come on with any degree of suddenness. Patients having very high blood sugar levels are quite ill, and symptoms will usually cause them to seek medical aid long before levels required to produce diabetic coma are reached. As a result these individuals are not up and about, seeking dental care. There is no necessity for a dental office to stock insulin as an emergency drug. Since the most rapidly acting insulin available has about a 2-hour latency period, it is hardly an emergency drug.

Adrenal insufficiency. The most common emergency occurring as the result of adrenal insufficiency is sudden hypotension or adrenal shock. This condition may occur in patients who have been taking steroid hormones for a period of time and who have the drug discontinued some time before a traumatic or stressful experience. This condition, termed *adrenal atrophy,* may persist for as long as a month after discontinuance of the medication. A similar condition, *adrenal exhaustion,* may occur following physically stressful situation (for example, debilitating diseases) that have been present for as little as 2 weeks.

In either adrenal atrophy or adrenal exhaustion the patient's ability to release endogenous steroid hormones in response to stressful situations is markedly reduced.

The emergency would be manifested as a sudden hypotensive episode much like that presented during an attack of syncope. In fact, differentiation between the two might be impossible. Proper positional changes coupled with airway maintenance and respiratory assistance must be applied if indicated.

Whereas the syncopal attack may usually be satisfactorily managed without drugs, adrenal shock nearly always requires the administration of vasopressors coupled with the administration of steroid hormones if the pressor effect is to be sustained. In the absence of steroid hormone administration the effect of vasopressor agents is short-lived.

Hydrocortisone (Solu-Cortef) or dexamethasone (Decadron) in 50 to 100 mg. and 4 to 12 mg. intravenous doses, respectively, will quickly rectify the episode.

SUMMARY

Measures have been described for the prevention, recognition, and treatment of systemic emergencies that may occur in the dental office. Emphasis is placed on the management of these emergencies without the use of drugs whenever feasible. It is my belief that, by far, the great majority of dental office emergencies may be satisfactorily managed without the use of any pharmacological agents. When the use of drugs is required in an emergency situation, they must invariably be coupled with proper attention to the mechanical steps described.

BIBLIOGRAPHY

Allen, G. D.: Dental anesthesia and analgesia, Baltimore, 1972, The Williams & Wilkins Co.

Beeson, P. B., and McDermott, W., editors: Cecil-Loeb textbook of medicine, ed. 13, Philadelphia, 1971, W. B. Saunders Co.

Bennett, C. R.: A clinical evaluation of fentanyl for outpatient sedation in dentistry, Oral Surg. **34:**880, 1972.

Bennett, C. R.: Monheim's general anesthesia in dental practice, ed. 4, St. Louis, 1974, The C. V. Mosby Co.

Bennett, C. R.: Monheim's local anesthesia and pain control in dental practice, ed. 6, St. Louis, 1978, The C. V. Mosby Co.

Collins, V.: Principles of anesthesiology, Philadelphia, 1970, Lea & Febiger.

Corbett, T. H., Cornell, R. G., Endres, J. L., and Millard, R. I.: Effects of low concentration of nitrous oxide on rat pregnancy, Anesthesiology **39:**299, 1973.

Corsen, G.: Neuroleptanalgesia and anesthesia: its usefulness in poor-risk cases, South. Med. J. **59:**801, 1966.

DiPalma, J. R., editor: Drill's pharmacology in medicine, ed. 4, New York, 1971, McGraw-Hill Book Co.

Foldes, F. F., Schapira, M., Torda, T. A., Duncolf, D., and Sniffman, H. P.: Studies on the specificity of narcotic antagonists, Anesthesiology **26:**320, 1965.

Foreman, P. A.: Pain control and patient management in dentistry-a review of current intravenous techniques, J. Am. Dent. Assoc. **80:**101, 1970.

von Frey, M.: Sachs Ges. Wiss. Math-Phys. Klin. (Ber.) **47:**166, 1895.

Gardocki, J. F., and Yelnosky, J.: A.: A study of some of the pharmacologic actions of fentanyl citrate, Toxicol. Appl. Pharmacol. **6:**48, 1964.

Goodman, L. S., and Gilman, A. Z.: The pharmacological basis of therapeutics: a textbook of pharmacology, toxicology, and therapeutics for physicians and students, ed. 4, New York, 1970, The Macmillan Co.

Guedel, A. E.: Signs, International Anesthesia Research Society Bull. No. 3, May, 1920.

Hershey, S. G., editor: Refresher courses in anesthesiology, vol. 3, Philadelphia, 1975, J. B. Lippincott Co.

King, C. H., and Stephen, C. R.: A new intravenous or intramuscular anesthetic, Anesthesiology **28:**258, 1967.

McCombs, R. P.: Fundamentals of internal medicine, ed. 4, Chicago, 1971, Year Book Medical Publishers, Inc.

Melzack, R., and Wall, P. D.: On the nature of cutaneous sensory mechanisms, Brain **85:**331, 1962.

Melzack, R., and Wall, P. D.: Pain mechanisms: a new theory, Science **150:**971, 1965.

Monheim, L. M.: Emergencies in the dental office. In Practical dental monographs, Chicago, 1963, Year Book Medical Publishers, Inc.

Mostery, J. W., Trudnowski, R. J., Seniff, A. M., Moore, R. H., and Case, R. W.: Clinical comparison of fentanyl with meperidine, J. Clin. Pharmacol. **8:**382, 1968.

Müller, J.: Elements of physiology, vol. 2, London, 1842.

Nafe, J. P.: In Murchison, C., editor: Handbook of general experimental psychology, Worcester, 1934.

Occupational disease among operating room personnel: a national study, Report of an Ad Hoc Committee on the Effects of Trace Anesthetics on the Health of Operating Room Personnel, Anesthesiology **41:**321, 1974

Oduntan, S. A.: Intravenous ketamine anesthesia, Anesthesia **25:**144, 1970.

Oral disease: target for the 70's, U.S. Department of Health, Education and Welfare, U.S. Public Health Service, National Institutes of Health, Washington, D.C., 1970, U.S. Government Printing Office.

Safar, P.: Cardiopulmonary resuscitation, a manual for physicians and paramedical instructors. Prepared for the World Federation of Societies of Anesthesiologists, 1968.

Safar, P.: Respiratory therapy, Philadelphia, 1968. F. A. Davis Co.

Sinclair, D. C.: Cutaneous sensation in the doctrine of specific energy, Brain **78:**584, 1955.

Stevens, W. C., Eger, E. I., II, White, A., Halsey, M. J., Munger, W., Gibbons, R. D., Dolan, W., and Shargel, R.: Comparative toxicities of halothane, isoflurane, and diethyl ether at subanesthetic concentrations in laboratory animals, Anesthesiology **42:**408, 1975.

Thomas, G. J., Pantalone, A. L., Buchanan, W. K., and Zeedick, J. F.: Summary of stages and signs in anesthesia, Anesth. Analg. **40:**43, 1961.

Venipuncture and venous cannulation, 97-0710/R2-75, Aug., 1972, Chicago, Abbott Laboratories.

Weddell, G., and Sinclair, D. C.: The anatomy of pain sensibility, Acta Neuroveg. (Wien) **7:**135, 1953.

GLOSSARY

absorption Passage of a substance into the interior of another by solution or penetration.

acapnia Diminished carbon dioxide in the blood.

acid Chemical substance that in aqueous solution undergoes dissociation with the formation of hydrogen ions (pH) ranging from 0 to 6.9.

acid salt Salt containing one or more replaceable hydrogen ions.

acidemia Decreased pH of the blood, irrespective of changes in the blood bicarbonate.

acidosis Acidemia or lowered blood bicarbonate with a tendency toward acidemia.

adrenergic Activated or transmitted by epinephrine or norepinephrine; a term applied to those fibers of the sympathetic system that liberate epinephrine or norepinephrine at a synapse when a nerve impulse passes.

adrenocortical steroid Hormone extracted from the adrenal cortex or a synthetic substance similar in chemical structure and biological activity to such hormones.

adrenolytic Term formerly used to denote a drug capable of blocking the effects produced by sympathetic nerve stimulation; the term *alpha-adrenergic* or *beta-adrenergic* blocking agent is more precise and should be used when appropriate.

adsorption Process believe to be physical in nature, in which molecules of a gas or liquid condense or adhere on the surface of another substance.

afferent Conveying from the periphery toward the center.

afferent impulse Impulse that arises in the periphery and is carried into the central nervous system; an afferent nerve conducts the impulse from the site of origin to the central nervous system.

airway Clear passageway for air into and out of the lungs; also a device for securing unobstructed respiration during general anesthesia or in states of unconsciousness.

alkali Strong water-soluble base.

alkaline reserve One of the buffer systems of the blood that can neutralize the acid valences formed in the body; it is made up by the base of weak acid salts and usually measured by determining the bicarbonate concentration of the plasma.

alkalosis Alkalemia or increased blood bicarbonate with a tendency toward alkalemia.

allergen Purified protein substance used to test a patient's sensitivity to foods, pollens, etc.

allergy Antigen-antibody reaction that results in a condition of unusual or exaggerated specific susceptibility to a substance that is harmless, in similar amounts, for the majority of members of the same species.

alpha-adrenergic blocking agent Drug that acts on alpha receptors, to block the vasoconstricting effect of epinephrine and norepinephrine.

alveolar ventilation Process of supplying alveoli with air or oxygen.

alveolus Air sac of the lungs, formed by terminal dilations of the brochioles.

analeptic Agent that acts to overcome depression of the central nervous system.

analgesia Loss of all pain sensation, caused by the administration of a drug, but without loss of consciousness.

analgesic (analgetic) Drug that raises the pain threshold.

analgetic drug (true) Drug that raises the pain threshold at a subcortical level; it should have no effect on cerebral cortical function.

anatomical dead space Actual capacity of the respiratory passages that extend from the nostrils to and include the terminal bronchioles.

anemic hypoxia Hypoxia brought about by the reduction of the oxygen-carrying capacity of the blood, as a result of the hemoglobin content or an alteration of the hemoglobin constituents.

anesthesia, basal State of narcosis, secured prior to the administration of a general anesthetic, which permits production of states of surgical anesthesia, with greatly reduced amounts of general anesthetic agents.

anesthesia, general Irregular and reversible depression of the cells of the higher centers of the central nervous system, making the patient unconscious and insensible to pain.

anesthetic agent Any drug capable of producing anesthesia.

anesthetic, local Drug that, when injected into the tissues, has little or no irritating effect and, when absorbed into the nerve, will temporarily interrupt the nerve's property of conduction.

anion Ion carrying a negative charge.

anoxia Condition of total lack of oxygen; frequently misused as a synonym for hypoxia.

anoxic hypoxia Hypoxia brought about by inadequate supply of oxygen in the inspired air or by interference with gaseous exchange in the lungs.

anticholinergic Drug that acts to block the effects of the neurohormone acetylcholine or of cholinergic drugs at postganglionic cholinergic neuroeffectors; a cholinergic-blocking agent.

anticholinesterase Drug that inhibits the enzyme cholinesterase, resulting in stimulation of organs innervated by cholinergic fibers.

antiemetic Drug used to prevent or relieve nausea and vomiting.

antihistaminic Drug that acts to prevent or antagonize the pharmacolgical effects of histamine and allergic symptoms that stem from the histamine released in the tissues.

antisialagogue Drug that reduces salivation.

apnea Temporary cessation of respiratory movements.

armamentarium Outfit of a practitioner or an institution, including books, medicines, and surgical supplies.

arrhythmia Any variation from the normal rhythm of the heart.

aseptic Not producing microorganisms; free from microorganisms.

asphyxia Condition of suffocation caused by restriction of oxygen intake plus interference with elimination of carbon dioxide.

asthma Disease marked by recurrent attacks of paroxysmal dyspnea, with wheezing, coughing, and a sense of constriction caused by the spasmodic contraction of the bronchi; it may result from direct irritation of the bronchial mucous membrane or from reflex irritation.

ataractic Capable of producing ataraxia.

ataraxia Calmness and complete peace of mind.

ataraxic Drug that produces calmness; a psychosedative.

atelectasis Complete collapse of a lung.

atom Smallest unit of an element that takes part in the formation of a compound; it consists of a positive nucleus surrounded by electrons.

augmentation Assistance to respiration by the application of intermittent pressure on inspiration.

base Solution that yields hydroxyl ions and neutralization in acid to form a salt and water; it is capable of combining with a protein; it turns red litmus paper blue and has a pH higher than 7.

basic salt Salt that contains replaceable or hydroxyl groups.

beta-adrenergic blocking agent Drug that acts on beta receptors to block sympathetic-induced vasodilation, cardiac acceleration, bronchiolar dilation, and hyperglycemia.

biotransformation Process whereby chemical agents undergo degradation and/or combination within the body, which usually renders the agent physiologically inactive; this term is not synonymous with detoxification, since an end product of biotransformation may be more toxic than the parent compound.

blood pressure Pressure of the blood on the walls of the arteries.

bradycardia Abnormal slowness of the heart (under 50 beats per minute) as evidenced by slowing of the pulse.

bradypnea Abnormal slowness of breathing.

bronchodilator Drug that dilates or expands the size of the lumina of the air passages of the lungs by relaxing the muscular walls.

bronchospasm Spasmodic contraction of the muscular coat of the bronchial tubes, such as occurs in asthma.

buffer Any substance in a fluid that tends to lessen the change in hydrogen ion concentration, which otherwise would be produced by adding acids or alkalies.

carbon dioxide absorber Device that removes carbon dioxide from a mixture of gases.

chemanesia Reversible amnesia produced by a chemical or drug.

Cholinergic blocking agent Drug that inhibits the action of acetylcholine or cholinergic drugs at postganglionic cholinergic neuroeffectors.

cholinergic drug Drug that mimics the effects of the neurohormone acetylcholine.

cholinesterase inhibitor Chemical that interferes with the activity of the enzyme cholinesterase.

compensated acidosis Condition in which the blood bicarbonate is usually higher than normal but the compensatory mechanisms have kept the pH within normal range.

compound Substance that consists of two or more chemical elements in union.

conduction Transfer of sound waves, heat, nerve influences, or electricity.

conjugation In chemistry, the joining of two compounds to produce another compound, such as the combination of a toxic product with some substance in the body to form a detoxified product, which is then eliminated.

conscious Being capable of rational response to a command and having all the protective reflexes intact, including the ability to maintain the airway in a patent state.

controlled respiration Maintenance of adequate pulmonary ventilation in apneic patients.

cough Sudden noisy expulsion of air from the lungs.

cyanosis Bluish tint to the skin.

degradation Reduction of a chemical compound to one that is less complex, as when groups (one or more) are split off.

depression Decrease of functional activity.

derivative Resultant of a chemical reaction.

detoxify (detoxicate) To remove the toxic quality of a substance.

dextrorotatory (dextrorotary) Rotating to the right.

diffusion Process of becoming widely spread, as when gases from a small jet spread throughout a room; in liquids the velocity of the molecules of two solutions will cause the molecules to diffuse, the diffusion varying in rate according to molecular weight and the temperature.

dose, lethal Amount of a drug that would prove fatal to the majority of persons.

dose, minimal lethal (MLD$_{50}$) Amount of a drug proving fatal to 50% of the animals in controlled experimental conditions.

dose, therapeutic Amount of a drug required to achieve the desired result; the amount will vary between minimal and maximal amounts.

dose, toxic Amount of a drug that causes untoward symptoms in the majority of persons.

drug Chemical agent that affects living protoplasm.

dyspnea Difficult, labored, or gasping respiration; inspiration, expiration, or both may be involved.

efferent Conveying impulses away from a nerve center toward the periphery.

efferent impulse Impulse that arises in the central nervous system and is carried to the peripheral nervous system; an efferent nerve conducts the impulse from the site of origin to the periphery.

element Simple substance that cannot be decomposed by chemical means; it is made up of atoms that are alike in their peripheral electronic configuration and chemical properties although differing in their nuclei, atomic weight, and radioactive properties.

emetic Drug that induces vomiting.

emphysema Presence of air in the intra-alveolar tissue of the lungs because of distention or rupture of the pulmonary alveoli with air; it may be interstitial (interlobular), when caused by the escape of air from the lungs into the interstitial tissue between the alveoli, or vesicular (alveolar), when caused by distention of the alveoli with air.

enzyme Substance elaborated by living cells and possessing catalytic properties.

esterase Enzyme that catalyzes the hydrolysis of an ester into an acid and an alcohol.

euphoric Substance that produces an exaggerated sense of well-being.

eupnea Easy or normal respiration.

exhalation valve Valve that permits escape of exhaled gases into the atmosphere and prevents their being rebreathed.

free nerve ending Peripheral terminal fiber of the sensory nerve.

full face mask Device used in anesthesia, which is placed over the nose and mouth and confines the anesthetic agents delivered into it and the respiratory tract to the nose and mouth.

ganglionic blocking agent Drug that prevents passage of nerve impulses at the synapse between preganglionic and postganglionic neurons.

gram Weight in the metric system, equal to 15.434 grains troy weight.

histotoxic hypoxia Hypoxia brought about by the inability of the tissue cells to use oxygen, which may be present in normal amount and tension.

hydrolysis Reaction between the ions of a salt and those of water to form an acid and a base, one or both of which are only slightly dissociated; a process whereby a large molecule is split by the addition of water; the end products divide the water, the hydroxyl group being attached to one and the hydrogen ion to the other.

hydroxyl Univalent radical that, in combination with other radicals, forms hydroxides.

hypalgesia Diminished sensation to pain, which results from a raised pain threshold.

hyperalgesia Greater than normal pain sensation that may be caused by a painful stimulus or a lowered pain threshold.

hypercapnia Presence of more than the normal amount of carbon dioxide in the blood, resulting from either an increase in carbon dioxide in the inspired air or a decrease in carbon dioxide elimination.

hyperpnea Increased respiratory volume, resulting from increased rate and depth of breathing.

hypertension Abnormally high blood pressure.

hypertonic Having a greater osmotic pressure than blood serum (said of a solution).

hypnotic Drug that induces sleep or depresses the central nervous system at the cortical level.

hypocapnia Deficiency of carbon dioxide in the blood.

hypopnea Abnormally shallow and rapid respirations.

hypotension Abnormally low tension, especially low blood pressure.

hypotensive agent Drug that reduces blood pressure, used in the treatment of hypertension.

hypoxemia Deficient oxygenation of the blood.

hypoxia Low oxygen content or tension.

idiosyncrasy Abnormal or unusual response; term used when an extremely small dose of a drug has been given; the reaction is similar to a toxic overdose.

impulse Uncontrollable wave of excitation, caused by a stimulus and transmitted along a nerve fiber.

injection Act of introducing a liquid into a part, such as the bloodstream or tissues.

insertion Act of implanting or, as in regional analgesia, of introducing the needle into the tissues.

ion Product formed by the electrolytic dissociation of a molecule; it carries one charge or more, positive or negative.

irritant Agent that causes irritation or stimulation.

irritation Act of stimulation; any condition of functional derangement and nervous irritability.

levorotatory (levorotary) Rotating to the left.

lipid Any one of a group of substances that include the fats and esters having analogous properties; lipids are organic substances—insoluble in water but soluble in alcohol, ether, and other fat solvents.

lipophilic Showing marked attraction to or solubility in lipids.

local anesthetic Drug that, when injected into tissue, has little or no irritating effect and, when absorbed into the nerve, will temporarily interrupt its conduction.

margin of safety Difference between lethal and toxic doses.

metabolism Sum of chemical changes involved in the function of nutrition; there are two phases—anabolism, constructive or assimilative changes, and catabolism, destructive or retrograde changes.

miotic Drug that constricts the pupil.

molecular weight Sum of atomic weights of all the atoms in a molecule.

molecule Chemical composition of two or more atoms that form a specific chemical substance.

mydriatic Drug that dilates the pupil.

myoneural blocking agent (skeletal muscle relaxant) Drug that prevents transmission of nerve impulses at the junction of the nerve and the muscle.

narcotic analgetic Drug that raises the pain threshold and depresses the cerebral cortex; it can induce euphoria.

narcotic antagonist Drug that acts specifically to reverse depression of the central nervous system produced by a narcotic analgetic.

nasal inhaler (nasal masks, nasal hood) Device used in anesthesia it is placed over the nose and confines the anesthetic agents delivered into it and the respiratory tract to the nose.

neutral solution Solution that has a pH of 7; equal numbers of hydrogen and hydroxyl ions are formed on dissociation.

noxious Hurtful, not wholesome.

orthopnea Inability to breathe except in an upright position.

oxidation (oxidization) Combination of oxygen with other elements to form oxides; the process in which an element gains electrons.

paralysis Loss or impairment of motor function.

parasympatholytic Drug that blocks nerve impulses passing from parasympathetic nerve fibers to postganglionic neuroeffectors.

parasympathomimetic Drug having an effect similar to that produced when the parasympathetic nerves are stimulated.

parenteral solution Sterile solution or substance prepared for injection.

partial pressure Pressure exerted by each of the constituents of a mixture of gases.

pH Concentration of hydrogen ions, expressed as the negative logarithm of base 10.

pKa Value equal to the pH at which 50% of the molecules are ionized.

polypnea Rapid or panting respiration.

potentiation Increase in the action of a drug caused by the addition of another drug that does not necessarily possess similar properties.

precipitate Insoluble solid substance that forms from chemical reactions between solutions.

pressor Drug that causes a rise in blood pressure.

propagation Reproduction or the continuance of an impulse along a nerve fiber in an afferent or an efferent direction.

psychomotor stimulant Drug that increases psychic activity, alertness, and motor activity.

psychosedative Calming agent that reduces anxiety and tension without depressing mental or motor function.

psychosomatic Pertaining to the mind-body relationship and producing bodily symptoms of a mental origin.

racemic Pertaining to a mixture of equal parts of a dextrorotatory and levorotatory compound.

radical Group of atoms that act as single elements when in chemical reactions.

reduction Removal of oxygen; addition of hydrogen; gain of electrons.

regional analgesia Reversible loss of pain sensation over an area of the body produced by blocking the afferent conduction of its innervation with a local anesthetic agent.

respiration Gaseous exchange betwen the cells of the body and its environment.

respiratory acidosis Acidemia produced by hypoventilation, which results in an increase in plasma carbonic acid and plasma bicarbonate.

respiratory alkalosis Alkalemia produced by hyperventilation; as a result of the plasma carbonic acid decreases and there is an excretion of bicarbonate in the urine to restore the carbonic acid–sodium bicarbonate ratio and prevent a change in pH; plasma bicarbonate is therefore decreased in respiratory alkalosis but raised in metabolic alkalosis.

salt Compound of a base and an acid; compound of an acid, some of whose replaceable hydrogen atoms have been substituted.

sedative Drug that allays excitement and slows the basal metabolic rate while producing only minor impairment of the cerebral cortex.

sialagogue Substance that increases the flow of saliva.

soporific Sleep-producing drug.

spasmolytic Drug that reduces spasm in smooth muscle.

stable Term applied to a substance that has no tendency to decompose spontaneously; in regard to chemical compounds, the term denotes their ability to resist chemical alterations.

stagnant hypoxia Hypoxia brought about by decreased circulation in an area.

sterile Being free from germ life.

stimulant Agent that causes an increase in functional activity, usually of the central nervous system.

stimulation Increased function of protoplasm, induced by some extracellular substance or agent.

stimulus Chemical, thermal, electrical, or mechanical influence that changes the normal environment of irritable tissue and creates an impulse.

strong acid Acid that is completely ionized in aqueous solution.

sympatholytic Term formerly used to describe a drug that blocked one of the effects of stimulation of the sympathetic nervous system; the term now more precisely refers to alpha-adrenergic blocking agents.

sympathomimetic Drug that partially or completely mimics the effects of sympathetic nerve stimulation or adrenal medullary discharge.

sympathoplegic Drug that blocks the action of sympathomimetic amines or limits sympathetic outflow.

synaptic conduction Conduction of a nerve impulse across a synapse.

synergism Ability of two drugs to increase the action of each other to an extent greater than a summation of the actions of each when used alone.

tachycardia Excessively rapid action of the heart; the pulse rate is usually above 100 beats per minute.

tachyphylaxis Decreasing response that follows consecutive injections at short intervals.

tachypnea Excessively rapid respiration; a respiratory neurosis marked by quick shallow breathing.

tranquilizer Nonmedical term for psychosedative.

uncompensated acidosis Acidemia usually accompanied by lowered blood bicarbonate, as after the ingestion of hydrochloric acid or in terminal nephritis. (In uncompensated carbon dioxide acidosis the bicarbonate may be normal.)

uncompensated alkalosis Alkalemia usually accompanied by an increased blood bicarbonate, as after the ingestion of sodium bicarbonate or after vomiting with the resultant loss of hydrochloric acid. (In uncompensated carbon dioxide alkalosis the bicarbonate may be normal.)

vagomimetic Drug with actions similar to those produced by stimulation of the vagus nerve.

vagovagal reflex Reflex in which the afferent impulses travel via the vagus nerve; the afferent impulses travel centrally via the sensory nucleus of the vagus; the efferent impulses travel centrally via the motor fibers of the vagus.

vasoconstrictor Agent that causes a rise in blood pressure by constriction of the blood vessels; in local areas there is constriction of the arterioles and capillaries.

vasodilator Agent that relaxes the smooth muscle walls of the blood vessels and increases their diameter.

vasopressor Agent that elevates blood pressure.

weak acid Acid that is only slightly ionized in aqueous solution.

INDEX